T0348633

Best Practices and Challenges to the Practice of Rheumatology

Editors

DANIEL J. WALLACE
R. SWAMY VENUTURUPALLI

RHEUMATIC DISEASE CLINICS OF NORTH AMERICA

www.rheumatic.theclinics.com

Consulting Editor
MICHAEL H. WEISMAN

February 2019 • Volume 45 • Number 1

ELSEVIER

1600 John F. Kennedy Boulevard • Suite 1800 • Philadelphia, Pennsylvania, 19103-2899
http://www.theclinics.com

RHEUMATIC DISEASE CLINICS OF NORTH AMERICA Volume 45, Number 1
February 2019 ISSN 0889-857X, ISBN 13: 978-0-323-65540-8

Editor: Lauren Boyle
Developmental Editor: Casey Potter

Rheumatic Disease Clinics of North America (ISSN 0889-857X) is published quarterly by Elsevier Inc., 360 Park Avenue South, New York, NY 10010-1710. Months of issue are February, May, August, and November. Business and editorial offices: 1600 John F. Kennedy Boulevard, Suite 1800, Philadelphia, PA 19103-2899. Periodicals postage paid at New York, NY and additional mailing offices. Subscription prices are USD 362.00 per year for US individuals, USD 706.00 per year for US institutions, USD 100.00 per year for US students and residents, USD 427.00 per year for Canadian individuals, USD 925.00 per year for Canadian institutions, USD 465.00 per year for international individuals, USD 925.00 per year for international institutions, and USD 230.00 per year for Canadian and foreign students/residents. To receive student/resident rate, orders must be accompanied by name of affiliated institution, date of term, and the *signature* of program/residency coordinator on institution letterhead. Orders will be billed at individual rate until proof of status received. Foreign air speed delivery is included in all *Clinics* subscription prices. All prices are subject to change without notice. **POSTMASTER:** Send address changes to *Rheumatic Disease Clinics of North America,* Elsevier Health Sciences Division, Subscription Customer Service, 3251 Riverport Lane, Maryland Heights, MO 63043. **Customer Service: 1-800-654-2452 (US and Canada). From outside of the US and Canada: 314-447-8871. Fax: 314-447-8029. For print support, e-mail: JournalsCustomerService-usa@elsevier.com. For online support, e-mail: JournalsOnline Support-usa@elsevier.com.**

Reprints. For copies of 100 or more of articles in this publication, please contact the Commercial Reprints Department, Elsevier Inc., 360 Park Avenue South, New York, New York, 10010-1710; Tel.: +1-212-633-3874, Fax: +1-212-633-3820, and E-mail: reprints@elsevier.com.

Rheumatic Disease Clinics of North America is covered in *MEDLINE/PubMed (Index Medicus), Current Contents/Clinical Medicine, Science Citation Index, ISI/BIOMED,* and *EMBASE/Excerpta Medica.*

Contributors

CONSULTING EDITOR

MICHAEL H. WEISMAN, MD
Cedars-Sinai Chair in Rheumatology, Director, Division of Rheumatology, Professor of Medicine, Cedars-Sinai Medical Center, Distinguished Professor, David Geffen School of Medicine at UCLA, Los Angeles, California, USA

EDITORS

DANIEL J. WALLACE, MD, FACP, MACR
Associate Director, Rheumatology Fellowship Program, Board of Governors, Professor of Medicine, Cedars-Sinai Medical Center, David Geffen School of Medicine, University of California, Los Angeles, Beverly Hills, California

R. SWAMY VENUTURUPALLI, MD, FACR
Clinical Associate Professor of Medicine, Cedars Sinai Medical Center, David Geffen School of Medicine, University of California, Los Angeles, Beverly Hills, California

AUTHORS

DANIEL F. BATTAFARANO, DO
Department of Medicine, San Antonio Military Medical Center, Fort Sam Houston, Texas

SULEMAN BHANA, MD
Rheumatologist, Crystal Run Health, Middletown, New York

JOEL A. BLOCK, MD
The Willard L. Wood, MD, Professor, Chair, Division of Rheumatology, Department of Internal Medicine, Rush University Medical Center, Chicago, Illinois

MARCY B. BOLSTER, MD
Division of Rheumatology, Allergy, and Immunology, Associate Professor of Medicine, Harvard Medical School, Director, Rheumatology Fellowship Training Program, Massachusetts General Hospital, Boston, Massachusetts

GERALD M. EISENBERG, MD, FACP, FACR
Director of Rheumatology, Illinois Bone and Joint Institute, Morton Grove, Illinois

THEODORE R. FIELDS, MD, FACP
Professor of Clinical Medicine, Weill Cornell College of Medicine, Attending Rheumatologist, Hospital for Special Surgery, New York, New York

JULIA A. FORD, MD
Division of Rheumatology, Brigham and Women's Hospital, Boston, Massachusetts

JON GLAUDEMANS
United Rheumatology, Hauppauge, New York

SOBIA HASSAN, MD, MRCP
Assistant Professor of Medicine, Division of Rheumatology, Rush University Medical Center, Chicago, Illinois

MEENAKSHI JOLLY, MD
Professor of Medicine and Behavioral Medicine, Fellowship Associate Program Director, Rush University Medical Center, Chicago, Illinois

ADAM KILIAN, MD
Division of Rheumatology, Department of Internal Medicine, University of Michigan, Ann Arbor, Michigan

CHRISTINE H. LEE, MD, MPH
Attending Physician, Cedars-Sinai Medical Center, Beverly Hills, California

SIAN YIK LIM, MD
Associate Professor of Medicine, Harvard Medical School, Director, Rheumatology Fellowship Training Program, Division of Rheumatology, Allergy and Immunology, Massachusetts General Hospital, Boston, Massachusetts

GOPIKA D. MILLER, MD
Health Sciences Assistant Clinical Professor, David Geffen School of Medicine, University of California, Los Angeles, Division of Rheumatology, Los Angeles Biomedical Research Institute, Harbor-UCLA Medical Center, Torrance, California

SEETHA U. MONRAD, MD
Division of Rheumatology, Department of Internal Medicine, University of Michigan, Ann Arbor, Michigan

KAREN MARIE MULLEN
CEO, NewView, Medical Consulting, LLC, Santa Clarita, California; Attune Health, Beverly Hills, California

KAREN BRANDT ONEL, MD
Professor of Pediatrics, Welll Cornell Medicine, Chief, Pediatric Rheumatology, Attending Physician, Hospital for Special Surgery, HSS Main Campus - Main Hospital, New York, New York

NORA G. SINGER, MD
Professor of Medicine and Pediatrics, Case Western Reserve University, Director, Division of Rheumatology, The MetroHealth System, Cleveland, Ohio

JASVINDER A. SINGH, MD, MPH
Professor of Medicine and Epidemiology, Endowed Professor, Musculoskeletal Outcomes Research, The University of Alabama at Birmingham School of Medicine, Birmingham, Alabama

MEGHAN M. SMITH, MHA
Administrator, Division of Rheumatology, Department of Internal Medicine, Rush University Medical Center, Chicago, Illinois

DANIEL H. SOLOMON, MD, MPH
Divisions of Rheumatology and Pharmacoepidemiology, Brigham and Women's Hospital, Boston, Massachusetts

PAUL SUFKA, MD
Rheumatologist, Regions Hospital & HealthPartners, St Paul, Minnesota

LAURA A. UPTON, MD
Georgetown University, School of Medicine, Washington, DC

R. SWAMY VENUTURUPALLI, MD, FACR
Clinical Associate Professor of Medicine, Cedars Sinai Medical Center, David Geffen School of Medicine, University of California, Los Angeles, Beverly Hills, California

DANIEL J. WALLACE, MD, FACP, MACR
Associate Director, Rheumatology Fellowship Program, Board of Governors, Professor of Medicine, Cedars-Sinai Medical Center, David Geffen School of Medicine, University of California, Los Angeles, Beverly Hills, California

Contents

In this article, we review the challenges and opportunities afforded by working in a government setting by providing the perspective of the Veterans Affairs experience as well as the county/public hospital experience from Los Angeles County Department of Health Services. This article highlights processes and services that are unique to practicing rheumatology in a government setting, specifically, resource allocation with clinic space and staffing; protocols for access to conventional and biologic disease modifying antirheumatic drugs; and research opportunities for rheumatologists working in a government setting. Our aim is to expand the reader's understanding of this practice setting.

Rheumatology has evolved rapidly over the past 20 years. The availability of numerous treatment interventions has dramatically altered patient outcomes and revitalized the specialty. At the same time, the economics of medical practice is challenging the practicing rheumatologist to seek more efficient and more attractive models of care delivery. These models of care must be attractive not only to rheumatologists and their patients but also to other interested parties as well, such as payers, government agencies, and accreditation bodies.

Pediatric rheumatology is an exciting and rewarding career area. However, challenges when attracting trainees to this field include practice often occurring in smaller groups compared with general pediatrics, available positions requiring relocation, and fluctuation in funding resulting in uncertainty regarding training positions. Having critical mass in pediatric divisions is important to ensure adequate mentoring and people power to produce scholarly work, reduce on-call frequency and mitigate faculty absences that result in unplanned addition of clinical work. Compensation has historically lagged behind that of general pediatrics. Increased research opportunities through organized networks, patient and parent engagement, and the increasing recognition of pediatric rheumatologists as contributing to scholarship has heightened the profile of pediatric rheumatology nationally and internationally.

Clinical trials evaluate the benefits and harms of medical interventions with the ultimate goal of establishing an evidence-based regimen that contributes to clinical decision making. Physicians benefit greatly from clinical research because it provides a greater understanding of epidemiology and health outcomes, and patients are given opportunities to participate in such trials. In this review, we discuss the challenges of conducting clinical trials investigating rheumatic diseases, including that of recruitment, finding the right trial, designing a budget, and performing a study in a timely manner. If done right, clinical investigation can be particularly rewarding both intellectually and financially.

Despite many effective treatments for gout, its management remains a challenge internationally. Options for optimizing gout management may differ in different practice sizes and settings. Gout incidence is rising and it continues to be associated with increased mortality. Education of patients and medical providers is essential, and newer gout medications need to be used in the most appropriate ways for cost-effective therapy. Special consideration needs to be given to such populations as the elderly and those with renal and cardiovascular disease in gout management. New agents are in development, which may add to the armamentarium for gout management.

RHEUMATIC DISEASE CLINICS OF NORTH AMERICA

SERIES OF RELATED INTEREST

Physical Medicine and Rehabilitation Clinics
https://www.pmr.theclinics.com/
Medical Clinics
https://www.medical.theclinics.com/
Primary Clinics: Clinics in Office Practice
https://www.primarycare.theclinics.com/
Dermatologic Clinics
Neurologic Clinics
https://www.neurologic.theclinics.com/

THE CLINICS ARE AVAILABLE ONLINE!
Access your subscription at:
www.theclinics.com

Foreword

Best Practices and Challenges to the Practice of Rheumatologists

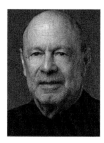

Michael H. Weisman, MD
Consulting Editor

This issue is a landmark in our series because it tries to address, in a scholarly documented way, the challenges we face every day in the world of Rheumatology science and practice from the physician perspective. In the carefully done article by Glaudemans, the current life-cycle shaping of rheumatology practice economics, with a focus on revenues, is very carefully described. The policies and practices of the major stakeholders: private and public insurance companies, pharmaceutical manufacturers, and pharmacy benefit managers (PBM), are enumerated as they impact the economics of rheumatology practice and the ultimate downstream effect on physician revenue. The role of rebates in shaping practice economics is discussed, along with the central role of payers in defining PBM policies. Glaudemans makes several suggestions to consider alternate value-based payment arrangements to sustain the model of private practice; these changes will require more careful attention paid to patient outcomes. The rheumatology shortage cycle is again facing our specialty and our patients with chronic diseases; Kilian and colleagues describe the impact of increasing numbers of retiring rheumatology specialists, more women entering the workforce, and rheumatology graduates seeking part-time employment. All these critical elements were identified by the 2015 workforce study group as the most significant factors driving the projected decline in supply of providers. Strategies to address the problem are described, but the solutions are necessarily going to be creative and, at times, expensive.

Hassan and colleagues discuss, very carefully, the challenges facing a career choice in academic medicine where expectations for performance have not been lessened or reduced in today's world. These current challenges are often no different from private practice, including physician burnout, less time caring (as opposed to documenting) for patients, and performing research that has an impact on our field. Miller and Singh review the challenges and opportunities facing employment as a rheumatologist in a

Rheum Dis Clin N Am 45 (2019) xiii–xiv
https://doi.org/10.1016/j.rdc.2018.10.002
0889-857X/19/© 2018 Published by Elsevier Inc.

government setting (county, VA) where the research opportunities and clinical commitments are often very rewarding on both a personal and a professional level. However, the caseload can be overwhelming, and it is important to recognize that the practice has unique features (space, staffing, referral patterns, and so forth), which must be recognized and appreciated. Jerry Eisenberg describes, in a highly personal way, the advantages to both patient and doctor when a physician-owned and directed multispecialty musculoskeletal group practice occurs and is well run in a community that appreciates the array of services in one setting. Singer and Onel discuss, in a highly thoughtful and appropriately well-documented way, how to sustain a successful pediatric rheumatology academic setting that addresses lifestyle issues (having a critical mass due to on-call issues and absences due to surrounding family life) as well as the need to connect with adult rheumatology research opportunities and collaborations.

Lee and Wallace describe, in sufficient detail, the multiplicity of challenges to perform therapeutic trials in an office setting. They point out that our diseases are quite complex with heterogenous patient populations; the issue of trust is adeptly discussed. In addition to recruitment challenges, these experienced trialists carefully identify some of the important logistical considerations to make the effort efficient and feasible. Karen Mullen, in a remarkably thoughtful article, describes the challenges of running an infusion center in a private practice from the often-neglected perspective of the patient: delivering care that is credible, effective, safe, and cost-effective. Ford and Solomon address a very important aspect of rheumatology patient care: the concept of a treatment-to-target (TTT) approach. Derived in Europe where it was robustly proven effective, there are unique challenges to implementing this TTT approach in our US health care systems, as discussed in this carefully documented article. Venuturupalli and colleagues address one of the most interesting and forward-thinking aspects of medical practice today: the discrepancy between the pace of digital medicine development versus its slow uptake in practice. Will better, safer, and less costly care translate into patient outcomes? The jury is still out. Lim and Bolster, very highly credible and successful educators and teachers themselves, have given us a beautifully documented article discussing the challenges (diverse lifestyles, multifaceted practice patterns, family obligations, and so forth) to optimizing medical learning and education in the long life span of today's practitioners. Finally, one would think that if we knew the cause and pathogenesis of a disease like gout it would cease to exist today. However, we know that this is not the case, and the very complex nature of managing gout patients in our diverse practice settings with differing alignments of patients and their doctors is thoughtfully discussed by Ted Fields in our last but not the least article.

Michael H. Weisman, MD
Director, Division of Rheumatology
Professor of Medicine
Cedars-Sinai Medical Center
8700 Beverly Boulevard
Los Angeles, CA 90048, USA

E-mail address:
Michael.Weisman@cshs.org

Preface

Best Practices and Challenges to the Practice of Rheumatologists

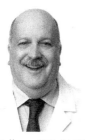   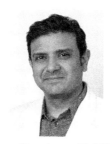

Daniel J. Wallace, MD, FACP, MACR   R. Swamy Venuturupalli, MD, FACR

Editors

Approximately 5000 rheumatologists in the United States treat over 100,000 patients every day. Despite 2.5 billion annual encounters, surprisingly little has been written regarding the subject. This issue of *Rheumatic Disease Clinics of North America* analyzes the impact of rheumatology practices by exploring how these hard-working subspecialty health care providers see patients in academic, office, group practice, government, and pediatric settings. Are the current practice models economically viable? How should the field strategize for future innovations and health care delivery systems? What are the roles for precision and personalized medicine? In this issue, 20 experts dissect and elucidate how our colleagues hone their craft and provide a framework for how rheumatology can remain a viable, innovative, and exciting field. We thank Dr Michael Weisman for his advice and wisdom and hope the reader can learn and potentially be empowered to make a difference, which benefits rheumatic disease patients and those who manage their care.

Daniel J. Wallace, MD, FACP, MACR
Cedars Sinai Medical Center
David Geffen School of Medicine
University of California–Los Angeles
8750 Wilshire Boulevard, Suite 350
Beverly Hills, CA 90211, USA

Rheum Dis Clin N Am 45 (2019) xv–xvi
https://doi.org/10.1016/j.rdc.2018.10.001
0889-857X/19/© 2018 Published by Elsevier Inc.

rheumatic.theclinics.com

R. Swamy Venuturupalli, MD, FACR
Cedars Sinai Medical Center
David Geffen School of Medicine
University of California–Los Angeles
8750 Wilshire Boulevard, Suite 350
Beverly Hills, CA 90211, USA

E-mail addresses:
danielwallac@gmail.com (D.J. Wallace)
drswamy@attunehealth.com (R.S. Venuturupalli)

The Economics of Rheumatology Practice in the United States

Jon Glaudemans

KEYWORDS

- Pharmacy benefit managers • Rebates • Biologics

KEY POINTS

- Private and public payer decisions—often implemented by pharmacy benefit managers (PBMs)—drive the revenues of rheumatology practices. Pharmaceutical manufacturers often pay substantial rebates to PBMs, which pass along some/most/all of the rebates to the relevant payers. PBMs impose a variety of mechanisms to shape physician prescribing decisions and are paid, in part, through rebates.
- Recently, 2 large payer-PBMs merged were announced: CVS Health seeks to purchase Aetna, and CIGNA intends to purchase Express Scripts. These mergers reflect the continued consolidation of payers and PBMs, but, given long-standing alignment of payer and PBM objectives, the mergers will not fundamentally alter the sources of the economic pressures facing rheumatology practices.
- Continued consolidation in private insurance, coupled with increasing scrutiny by Medicare, will continue to squeeze rheumatologists' ability to be compensated for managing high-cost chronically ill patients on a fee-for-service or buy-and-bill basis. Relief from these economic pressures and forces may require rheumatologists to consider value-based payment arrangements, which will require careful attention to managing and measuring patient outcomes, and, in some payment models, to develop and manage physician-led formularies.

As described in the balance of this volume's articles, rheumatologists face a series of challenges to their ability to treat patients, advance the standard of care, improve the health of their communities, and, importantly, to achieve these goals in an economically sustainable fashion. Using net compensation to the average rheumatologist as one measure of economic sustainability, the annual Medscape survey of physician compensation reveals that the average 2018 compensation for a rheumatologist is $257,000—approximately 78% of the average $329,000 compensation for all specialists and approximately 9% above the comparable 2017 figure.[1]

Disclosure: J. Glaudemans is CEO of United Rheumatology, a for-profit provider of management and information services to independent rheumatologists. He reports no other financial conflicts of interest.
United Rheumatology, 150 Motor Parkway, Suite 108E, Hauppauge, NY 11788, USA
E-mail address: jonglaudemans@unitedrheumatology.org

Rheum Dis Clin N Am 45 (2019) 1–12
https://doi.org/10.1016/j.rdc.2018.09.001
0889-857X/19/© 2018 Elsevier Inc. All rights reserved.

rheumatic.theclinics.com

Rheumatology practice revenues derive from several sets of services:

- Payments for professional services, including office visits and patient counseling
- Payments for ancillary services, such as diagnostic imaging, laboratory, drawing lab specimens and interpreting results research studies, and related services
- Payments for the delivery and management of physician-administered medications

Total compensation is revenue net of expenses, whether received or incurred by a solo practice, a group practice, a hospital-based practice, or by institutional sponsors.

In most settings, practice revenues are calculated on a fee-for-service basis: each price for each service is contracted for, and providing more services generates more revenue. Some practices also participate in value-based payment (VBP) arrangements, accountable care organizations, and various pilots and demonstrations, where revenues may accrue outside of the fee-for-service category, such as risk-sharing revenues (or costs).

For the first 2 categories— professional and ancillary services— most revenue arrangements are established simply and solely between the physician/practice and the payer. In some cases, such as clinical trials, the revenue arrangements vary by trial.

In the third category—physician-administered drugs—the rheumatology practice operates at the bottom of a long and complex distribution system of stakeholders, including (1) payers, (2) manufacturers, and, (3) pharmacy benefit managers (PBMs). The eventual revenue to a rheumatology practice for administering these complex and costly medications depends largely on the decisions made within and across these 3 stakeholders.

This article examines these 3 major sets of stakeholders and their role on the economics of the rheumatology practice. Although other stakeholders with discernible impact on the flow of funds to rheumatology practices exist—including wholesalers, specialty pharmacies, group purchasing organizations, and so forth—the primary drivers of rheumatology practice revenues are decisions made by and among payers, manufacturers, and PBMs.

In **Fig. 1**, the relationships between these 4 stakeholders are summarized. Below, we examine these various stakeholders' decision-making incentives and goals as they relate to the economics of the rheumatology practice. This article begins by describing the various payers' roles in shaping the economic environment for rheumatology practices. Then, after a discussion of the manufacturers' impact on practice economics, the article examines how PBMs play a pivotal role connecting payers and manufacturers and thus help shape a practice's economics for physician-administered drugs, which for many provides important supplemental income to the core professional and ancillary revenue streams strike balance of sentence, is examined.

This 2018 characterization of the US health care ecosystem will continue to evolve in the years ahead. A decade ago, the various relationships, incentives, and pressures (described later) were markedly different; readers should recognize that, as in medicine and science, the design of the health care market continues to advance, albeit not always to the benefit of the patient and physician.

PAYERS: MAKERS OF THE GOLDEN RULES

This discussion beings with relationship between a patient and the public or private payer who compensates the doctor or hospital and/or pays for the prescribed drug.

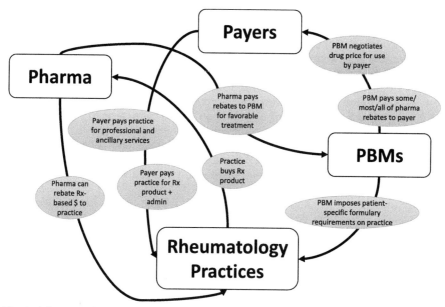

Fig. 1. Schematic diagram of rheumatology practice revenue ecosystem. Pharma, Manufacturer of Drug Therapy; Rx, Prescription Therapy; $, Dollars.

To steal a phrase, those with the gold make the rules, and the rules are set by the payer, who uses premiums paid by a group of individuals and assumes financial liability for the cost of health care for that group of individuals. The rules include which services or products are paid for in which settings of care, the amounts paid for services and products, and whether additional clinical or financial review is required prior to payment, among others. In the US health care system, most of these rules are set implicitly or explicitly by 1 of 5 main sets of payers: Employers; Medicare; Medicaid; Marketplaces; and the uninsured. A sixth category of coverage provides payments for care delivered to military servicemembers, veterans, and their families. This unique set of insurance programs is beyond the scope of this review (**Table 1**).

Most Americans Obtain Their Health Insurance Directly or Indirectly Through Their Employer

Most employers pay most of the cost of employees' health insurance, often referred to as employer-sponsored insurance (ESI).[2] Large employers generally offer their

Table 1
Health insurance coverage in the United States: 2016

	Employer	Individual	Medicare	Medicaid	Military	Uninsured	Total
Number covered during 2016 (millions)	178.5	52.0	53.4	62.3	14.6	28.0	320.3

Note: Numbers do not add to total, given multiple sources of coverage in a year.
  Total represents US population.
  Data from Barnett JC, Berchick ER. Current population reports, P60-260, health insurance coverage in the United States: 2016. Washington, DC: U.S. Government Printing Office; 2017. Available at: https://www.census.gov/content/dam/Census/library/publications/2017/demo/p60-260.pdf. Accessed July 15, 2018.

employees reasonably generous coverage options and usually self-insure the risk of providing insurance to their employees. Under federal law, large employers can create a system of benefits applicable to all of their employees regardless of state of residence. By self-insuring, the large employer is choosing to bear most or all of the actuarial risk of providing a promise of insurance coverage to their employees. If actual costs exceed expected costs, the large employer picks up the tab. Many large employers engage private insurance companies on an a la carte basis to provide administrative services like paying claims and tracking expenses.

Smaller employers, who often lack the size and cash reserves to accurately predict expenses or, in the previous case, to cover a shortfall, generally engage a private insurance company to bear the risk and define the benefits for the small employer's employees.

In both cases, and of interest to rheumatology patients and physicians and their keen interest in the cost and availability of biologic medications, both large risk-bearing employers and private insurers of small employers tend to contract with PBMs to assist in administering and managing payments for prescription drugs. As discussed in more detail later, the specific policies adopted by PBMS—formularies, prior authorization, step edits, and so forth—arise entirely from payers' and employers' demands for strategies to manage their drug spending.

Many large employers work with their PBM to create a customized formulary, where a large company contracting with a particular PBM may prefer 1 drug in a class, and another large employer, contracting with the same PBM, may prefer another drug in a class. In some cases, the large employer chooses simply to implement the PBM's standard formulary. Adding to the complexity, small employers' insurance companies may also choose to deploy a variety of formularies.

A single rheumatology practice is forced to navigate a variety of benefit designs and often dozens of employer-specific formularies, many of which may be administered by the same PBM and which may apply inconsistent formulary policies for the same medicine, depending on the patient's employer. Ultimately, the ESI plans, and their contracted PBMs, determine how much a physician is paid, which drugs the physician can prescribe, and under which coverage conditions (prior authorization, step edits, and so forth). These formularies usually result in rebates being paid by the manufacturer to the PBM and the payer.

Employers and their insurance company partners share a common perspective on the economics of health care: meet the employee workforce's demand for high-quality, easily-accessed, and inexpensive health care at a price affordable to the employer or a premium acceptable to the private insurer. Clearly, tradeoffs are required: offer skimpy benefits—high employee cost-sharing, narrow networks, and so forth —and risk losing a competitive benefits package to attract employees. Offer rich benefits—no cost-sharing, open networks, and so forth—and reduce profits or lose market share establish generous payment schedules for physicians' professional services and expand the managed care network, only to see reduced profits; pay specialists too little, and risk employee dissatisfaction. In every case, including the use of formularies, the payer is motivated to toe the line between too much and too little.

More generally, payers are now marketing insurance benefits where patients have little or no first-dollar coverage, and instead choose to pay a lower premium in exchange for agreeing to pay a high deductible. Often coupled with federally qualified health savings accounts, these high-deductible plans[3] require patients to be personally liable for 100% of their health cost up to a predefined maximum. As discussed later, the use of rebates and formularies has created a spread in the difference between the list price of the drug and the net price. For individuals in high-deductible plans, the plan often requires the patient to pay the list price; once the deductible is met, the payer reverts to the net price for payment calculations.

For rheumatologists, the PBMs hired by employers and insurance companies are efforts to provide just enough access to expensive products at an affordable price…for employers and insurers, and, arguably, for patients as well. Rheumatologists' frustration with PBM rules, regulations, and formularies must recognize the underlying motivation of the PBM-engaging employer or insurer, where the payer ultimately sets the overall balance between access, quality, and cost in every health care transaction. Later, PBMs are discussed in more detail, and some of the economic incentives and relationships between employers, payers, and PBMs are untangled.

Medicare Is the Insurer for Most Americans over the Age of 65

Simplifying, Medicare consists of 4 separate, intersecting programs, each with its own set of rules and regulations:

- Part A, setting rules and making payments for hospital services
- Part B,[4] setting rules and making payments for physician services, including payments for physician-administered drugs as are typical in a rheumatologist's practice
- Part C, setting rules and making payments to Medicare Advantage (MA) insurance companies, who take a fixed sum from Medicare and then bear the insurance risk to pay for care delivered to those Medicare beneficiaries who make the annual voluntary choice to join an MA plan
- Part D,[5] setting rules and making payments to private insurance companies who have agreed to provide prescription drug coverage for self-administered drugs to eligible Medicare beneficiaries. Within the Part D program, the benefit design is such that some beneficiaries are liable for the full cost of a drug within a defined coverage gap. How the growing spread between drugs' list and net prices has an impact on patients inside the coverage gap is discussed later.

Because Medicare is the single largest single payer of health care services in the United States, its policies—including audit and compliance requirements—have a significant impact on the economics of rheumatology practices. The specific rules within each of the Medicare programs—A, B, C, and D—use differing payment models for services and drugs needed to treat many patients seen by rheumatologists.

For drugs administered by physicians, Part B pays the physician for the service, and, for the drug, reimburses the physician for the acquisition cost of the drug and a percentage add-on to recognize the role played by the office in purchasing and administering the product. Patients make a modest copayment for Part B drugs. For self-administered drugs, the private Part D plans make no payment to the physician, and patient copayments tend to be significantly higher than those for Part B drugs. Periodically, Medicare tries to reconcile these different payment models, with their differing demands on patients' pocketbooks. For patients in a Part C MA plan, the same B versus D distinction tends to obtain: payments for physician-administered drugs are paid by the private MA plan to the physician, and most MA plans use or are licensed as a Part D plan.

The rheumatology practice with the usual mix of pre-Medicare and post-Medicare patients often faces patient pressure to begin or continue the physician-administered products, because their financial liability is lower in Part B. Conversely, Medicare's trust fund spends less on Part D products (because patients pay more), so the incentive of the payer, in this case, is to shift the patient to a self-administered product. Over the past decade, after the introduction of Part D, Medicare policymakers in Congress and the administration continue to seek reductions in the growth rate of Medicare, often using a mix of payment reductions and efforts to create more efficient models of care and payment.

Looking ahead, rheumatology practices with a critical mass of Medicare beneficiaries (or whose patient cohorts are aging into Medicare), will face continued downward pressure on their revenues associated with evaluation and management services,[6] as part of secular federal budgetary pressures affecting all specialists, as well as continued disruptive proposals and policies in the Part B and D drug reimbursement spaces. Given that many rheumatologists or their sponsoring institutions earn significant revenue from the Part B drug payments, continued monitoring and vigilance in this space are warranted.

Medicaid Is the Public Insurer for Many Americans with Low Incomes

Under a federal-state partnership, all states provide a minimum insurance benefit to some or most of their low-income residents.[7] This insurance coverage is ultimately provided by the state, but most states have delegated the day-to-day functions to private managed care companies operating under state license. The coverage rules vary slightly by state, and many states have chosen to expand their eligibility criteria to include the near-poor under the terms of the Affordable Care Act.

For the most part, states' Medicaid reimbursement rates for visit and procedure codes are substantially below Medicare rates, much less commercial rates. This is true whether the state pays the provider directly or through a managed care intermediary. States' budgets are driven almost entirely by their education and Medicaid commitments, and continued revenue and tax pressures on states limit the possibility of any economic relief for rheumatology services provided to Medicaid patients.

Marketplace-Based Coverage Is Available to Everyone, with Subsidies for Those with Moderate Incomes

Created by the Affordable Care Act, Marketplace coverage is the term-of-art for a set of standardized insurance plans offered under the ACA through Federal or State-run "Marketplace" where individuals can compare coverage and premiums of approved plans.[8] These plans are presented to individuals and small employers via governmentally sponsored online Marketplaces. These plans' minimum benefits are governed by statute and resemble the coverage offered by small employers directly by private insurers. Most individuals obtaining coverage in their own right obtain their coverage through the Marketplaces.

Even more so than ESI-based plans, Marketplace-participating payers face the same pressures to offer the right balance of quality, access, and cost. Given the Marketplace's attraction to moderate income individuals, Marketplace plans compete largely on who can deliver the minimal required benefits for the lowest premium. In general, the relevant benefit, network, and coverage rules for a state are the ceiling, and plans compete on premium—by keeping provider payments lower and networks narrower than in many ESI plans.

As a result, rheumatology practices are not likely to experience significant increases in fee-based compensation levels for seeing Marketplace plan members/patients. It may be possible that, as addressed elsewhere in this issue, the growing imbalance of supply and demand for rheumatology services may result in upward rate pressure on insurers—whether ESI or Marketplace. Insurers and employers, however, are historically slow to respond to such imbalances, especially if the specialty tends to manage high-cost (ie, less-profitable/more-expensive) patients.

Some Americans Cannot Afford Insurance or Cannot or Choose Not to Purchase Insurance

Approximately 10% of Americans do not have health insurance.[9] Some are able to afford insurance but choose not to purchase coverage; others cannot afford insurance. Still others are undocumented residents, who may fear the repercussions of purchasing private or public insurance. In all cases, these patients are asked to pay cash for services. Given the expense of many of the medications routinely prescribed by rheumatologists, these cash-paying patients pose a special challenge to the economics of a diverse rheumatology practice.

Summary—the payer wants more for less

The private employers, private insurers, and public programs that pay for care set the economic framework for the rheumatology practice. Not surprisingly, each payer wants more for less. To achieve this goal, private and public payers have to date largely relied on managing the fee schedules for professional and ancillary rheumatology services, and many have developed specialty-focused quality-improvement and cost-reduction initiatives and programs, many of which have an impact on the rheumatologist. Payers have also developed a series of wide-range strategies and programs to manage the third category of rheumatology practice revenues: payments associated with the administration of expensive medications to treat rheumatology patients.

As referenced previously, many payers rely on PBMs to address the cost of medications. To understand the impact these PBMs have on the economics of the rheumatology practice, the role of the manufacturer must first be addressed and the basis for the formation and evolution of PBMs as a response to payer needs and demands described.

PHARMA: DELIVERER AND PURVEYOR OF THE GOLDEN EGGS

The advent of biologics to treat patients with rheumatologic diseases has improved the lives of millions of people and, as well, heralded a new economic environment for practicing rheumatologists. It is beyond the scope of this article or issue to discuss the economics of pharmaceutical innovation, research and development (R&D), and, ultimately, product pricing. It is enough to acknowledge that innovator companies take risk on basic R&D and expect returns commensurate with the risk. Other pharmaceutical companies focused on purchasing preapproval pipeline products or marketing approved products also expect returns commensurate with the market's assessment of risk. Thus, once approved, the patent holder of the market-approved product approved biosimilar has a strong economic incentive to maximize their revenues (short/long-term) from sales of their product.

Drug revenues depend in part on the volume of units sold as well as the net revenue per unit sold. Importantly, volume is usually related to efficacy of a product: the better it works, the more it is used. It is also true that effective marketing of an effective product yields higher sales than ineffective marketing of an (equally) effective product, and the advantage of first arrival on the subsequent market should also be recognized. The rheumatologist influences the volume of product sold though her prescribing decisions, with many of these decisions influenced or directed by the payer-sponsored, PBM-developed formulary and rebate strategies, discussed later. One of the implications of the payer-PBM approach to using rebates and formularies to shape price and quantity is the "gross-to-net" distinction between list price paid by some (cash patients) and used to calculate coinsurance and deductible responsibilities, and the net price paid by the insurer.

A Manufacturer's List Price for Its Product Bears Only a Loose Relationship to the Manufacturer's Net Revenue/Unit

Manufacturers set an original price — what they charge — for their product, and, after many arms-length transactions between wholesalers, distributors, pharmacies, insurers, and physicians, eventually record a per-product revenue — The difference between the gross price and the net price is often significant, and can be referred to as the "gross-to-net" bubble what they receive — that is, significantly less than the original price. Without dwelling on the complex concepts of Wholesale Acquisition Cost, Average Sales Price, 340B Pricing, Medicaid Best Price, and so forth, the existence of gross-to-net difference between price and revenue impact on the economics of rheumatology practice (**Table 2**).

As discussed previously, in separate 2017 reports, 2 large R&D-based pharmaceutical manufacturers reported their average increase in list prices, and their average increase in net realized price. The dynamic of the growing wedge between gross price and net price has been well-tracked and documented by several observers, notably Adam Fein and his informative blog, www.drugchannels.net.[10] The data indicate a growing gap between the list price and the net price.

Below the reported gross and net price increases, the table shows the growth of a hypothetical product with $100 million in sales in 2012. Although rebate-formulary dynamics predate the first year in these tables, in the example, from that $100 million base, both companies instituted average list prices increases that would have, if undiscounted, resulted in 2017 sales of approximately $152 million and $187 million by 2017. Instead, because of discounts, rebates, and other payments to the payers, PBMs, and other distribution system stakeholders, the actual revenues in this hypothetical example were only $112M and $135M, respectively. for a drug.

The difference — $40 million and $52 million — represents the "gross-to-net bubble". Because the contractual arrangements between payers, PBMs, and manufacturers are confidential, the disposition of this "gross-to-net bubble" is unknown, but likely results in revenues accruing to both PBMs and payers.

With Fein estimating the financial size of this gross-to-net bubble at $150 billion in 2017, it is fair to ask the question: Where did the money go? For that, the role of PBMs needs to be understood. For the practicing rheumatologist and the patient, the rebate-formulary strategy and the "gross-to-net bubble" are 2 sides of the same coin. With formularies driving clinical decisions, and with patients liable for list prices in many circumstances, understanding practice economics requires looking at the other side of the coin — formularies and rebates.

PHARMACY BENEFIT MANAGERS: THE GOLD BEHIND THE CURTAIN

As discussed previously, payers want more for less. To achieve this in the traditional physician and hospital settings, payers establish coverage rules (what they will pay for under what circumstances), payment rules (how much they will pay for a product or service), and preferred relationships with participating physicians and hospitals (who they will pay) as well as track results (clinical and economic). Until the late 1980s, many of these companies treated the coverage and payment for prescription drugs in 1 of 2 ways: either drugs were not covered or, more likely, they were treated as "just another insurance benefit."

In the early 1990s, payers began to take note of the rising price of small-molecule medicines, the emergence of expensive large-molecule biologics, and the increased number of medications available to treat a given disease. Not surprisingly, payers began to adopt many of the same strategies used to manage physician and hospital benefits: limit coverage to certain drug therapies; structure payments that extract

Table 2
Select manufacturer-reported growth in average list and net prices, 2013–2017

	Year-to-Year Increase						Illustrative Growth of 100 Million in 2012 Revenues $						2013–2017 Growth
	2012	2013	2014	2015	2016	2017	2012	2013	2014	2015	2016	2017	
Janssen (A)													
List price	NA	9.0%	8.3%	9.7%	8.5%	8.1%	100.0	109.0	118.0	129.5	140.5	151.9	139%
Net revenue	NA	4.8%	2.5%	5.2%	3.5%	−4.6%	100.0	104.8	107.4	113.0	117.0	111.6	106%
Rebates, etc.	NA	4.2%	5.8%	4.5%	5.0%	12.7%	0.0	4.2	10.6	16.5	23.5	40.3	960%
Lilly (B)													
List price	NA	15.0%	11.8%	16.3%	14.0%	9.7%	100.0	115.0	128.6	149.5	170.5	187.0	163%
Net revenue	NA	11.9%	1.6%	9.4%	2.4%	6.0%	100.0	111.9	113.7	124.4	127.4	135.0	121%
Rebates, etc.	NA	3.1%	10.2%	6.9%	11.6%	3.7%	0.0	3.1	14.9	25.1	43.1	52.0	1677%

Data from Janssen 2017 U.S. Transparency report. Available at: http://jnj-jansen.brightspotcms.com/us/us-pharmaceutical-transparency-report/pricing-and-patient-access. Accessed July 15, 2018; and Eli Lilly and Company, 2017 integrated summary report. Available at: https://www.lilly.com/2017-integrated-summary-report. Accessed July 15, 2018.

lower prices for higher volumes; and, more recently, create preferred relationships with pharmacies.

Formularies[11]—and their associated clinical and economic review processes—have long been used by physician and hospital groups to help prescribers choose the appropriate medicine for their patient. Over time, payers began to adapt the processes used inside clinical settings and created mechanisms to create a marketplace for drug manufacturers to present a product-price-value proposition to the payer, arguing for coverage. In many therapeutic classes, where the scientific and clinical literature suggested equal efficacy between 2 or more competing products, payers saw a chance to repeat their preferred relationship strategy already used with physicians and hospitals. In both arenas, the payers offered higher volumes (visits, admissions, and drug sales) in exchange for lower prices. Manufacturers began to offer lower prices in exchange for more attractive coverage and payment rules.

Unlike the markets for physician and hospital services, however, the ability of manufacturers and payers to agree on a price is constrained by significant regulation, where public policies seek to make drugs more affordable to low-income individuals (so-called Medicaid Best Price[12]) and those hospitals that treat a disproportionate number of these patients (so-called 340B Hospitals[13]). These regulatory considerations effectively linked the prices offered to a private payer with prices paid by the public payer. To maintain the distinction, and simplifying greatly, the nature of the manufacturer-payer price-for-volume agreements became more dependent on creative rebate and charging arrangements that maintain a degree of separation between the private and public worlds. As discussed previously, these creative arrangements increasingly drove a widening gross-to-net pricing bubble, with implications for patients and physicians.

Although this bubble has implications for patients, the day-to-day requirements imposed by PBMs – to enforce their volume commitments to the manufacturers – on physician prescribing behaviors has the more direct impact on the economics of the rheumatology practice. Over the past 15 years or so, PBMs, working with their payer sponsors, have introduced a wide array of formulary management tools that have an impact on practice economics.

PBM formulary development tends to begin by sorting drugs into therapeutic classes—grouping drugs that treat one condition into a single class. Based on clinical and economic input, the PBM usually offers the manufacturers of a class's drugs the chance to proffer a price—or, more usually, a gross-to-net combination, with rebates. All other things being equal (and they rarely are), the PBM has an incentive to choose the drug with the lowest net price to the PBM and/or payer and to give it preferential coverage in the formulary. Often, there are clinical or market considerations that lead to more than one preferred drug in a class.

Once the formulary design is established within a class, the PBM often adopts a series of compliance requirements to assure that physicians prescribe consistently with the PBM-determined preferences. In this way, the manufacturer can be assured that the pricing concessions offered during the formulary negotiation result in the expected volume of sales (having traded price for quantity).

These compliance requirements often include require the physician to obtain so-called prior authorization from the PBM prior to prescribing a particular product as well as requirements that PBM- preferred drugs are tried before less preferred drugs. Each of these requirements imposes administrative burdens on the rheumatology office—and collectively, the use of formularies and their associated compliance requirements not only dictates the clinical decisions of physicians but also imposes considerable practice expense loads on the physician.

Rheumatologists are more aware than many other specialties of these rules and impositions. It is easy to blame the PBMs for these new rules, but the payer—the original public or private insurer—is the real driver behind formularies. Facing a world of many new and emerging therapies with often uncertain clinical implications and rising costs, payers delegated a tried-and-true strategy to get more for less: trade promises of higher volume for lower prices. Other PBM services—medication compliance, generic substitution, and others—all followed the initial payer delegation of accountability to the PBM to deliver more for less.

For the rheumatology practice whose economics and patients are impacted by the efforts of payers and PBMs, there seem to be 2 pathways out of the gross-to-net/formulary-rebate wilderness:

- One path involves the pursuit of VBP approaches with payers and manufacturers, where physicians play a central role in delivering more for less, perhaps by assuming the responsibility of selecting the most clinically effective —and most cost-effective—therapy for a patient. In these VBP models, payers, physicians, and patients tend to share in the savings associated with more cost-effective care.
- A second path involves accepting the practice of the continued imposition of payer-based, PBM-driven formulary rules and related pricing inefficiencies, with any savings tending to accrue to the payer and/or the PBM.

For the former pathway, the small size of most rheumatology practices suggests the need for rheumatologists to align with hospitals or professional organizations that can create economies of scale and develop VBPs. For the latter pathway, the future is already being written: in the last year, 2 of America's largest payers—Aetna[14] and Cigna[15]—have announced plans to merge with 2 of America's largest PBMs—CVS and Express Scripts. Without rheumatology-based and rheumatology-led VBP models, it is safe to say that combined payer-PBM limits on prescribing will persist. Conversely, the emergence of physician-led VBP models, coupled with growing consumer frustration with the gross-to-net bubble and the formulary-rebate parlay, could result in more rheumatology practices choosing another approach to the 'more for less' imperative.

REFERENCES

1. Available at: https://www.medscape.com/slideshow/2018-compensation-overview-6009667#3. Accessed July 15, 2018.
2. See health insurance: a primer, congressional research service. United States Library of Congress; 2015. Available at: https://www.everycrsreport.com/files/20150108_RL32237_5ec7ab29996bb919f1ab1be6e7c1460b2a01295c.pdf. Accessed July 15, 2018.
3. Health savings accounts and high deductible health plans grow as valuable financial planning tools" issue brief, America's Health Insurance Plans (AHIP), 2018. Available at: https://www.ahip.org/2017-survey-of-health-savings-accounts/. Accessed July 18, 2018.
4. Part B Drugs Payment Systems, U.S. Congress Medicare Payment Advisory Committee (MedPAC) Research Brief. 2017. Available at: http://medpac.gov/docs/default-source/payment-basics/medpac_payment_basics_17_partb_final.pdf?sfvrsn=0. Accessed July 15, 2018.

5. Part D payment system, U.S. Congress Medicare Payment Advisory Committee (MedPAC)Research Brief. 2017. Available at: http://medpac.gov/docs/default-source/payment-basics/medpac_payment_basics_17_partd_final86a411adfa9c665e80adff00009edf9c.pdf?sfvrsn=0. Accessed July 15, 2018.

6. Centers for Medicare and Medicaid Services, CMS proposes historic changes to modernize medicare and restore the doctor-patient relationship. 2018. Available at: https://www.cms.gov/Newsroom/MediaReleaseDatabase/Press-releases/2018-Press-releases-items/2018-07-12.html. Accessed July 23, 2018.

7. Medicaid Physician Payment Policy – Issue Brief, Medicaid and CHIP Payment and Access Commission (MACPAC). 2016, Available at: https://www.macpac.gov/wp-content/uploads/2016/04/Medicaid-Physician-Payment-Policy.pdf. Accessed July 18, 2018. See also: Medicaid: A Primer, U.S. congress congressional research service. 2012. Available at: https://fas.org/sgp/crs/misc/RL33202.pdf. Accessed July 18, 2018.

8. "Overview of health insurance exchanges," U.S. Congress Congressional Research Service. 2018. Available at: https://fas.org/sgp/crs/misc/R44065.pdf. Accessed July 15, 2018.

9. Federal subsidies for health insurance coverage for people under age 65: 2018-2028, Congress of the United States. Congressional Budget Office; 2018. Available at: https://www.cbo.gov/system/files?file=2018-06/53826-health insurancecoverage.pdf. Accessed July 18, 2018.

10. "The gross-to-net bubble topped $150 Billion in 2017," Adam Fein. 2018. Available at: https://www.drugchannels.net/2018/04/the-gross-to-net-rebate-bubble-topped.html. Accessed July 18, 2018.

11. Formulary management: issue brief, academy of managed care pharmacy. 2009. Available at: http://www.amcp.org/WorkArea/DownloadAsset.aspx?id=9298. Accessed July 18, 2018.

12. Medicaid best price: prescription drug pricing policy brief. Ramsey Baghdadi, Health Affairs; 2017. Available at: https://www.healthaffairs.org/do/10.1377/hpb20171008.000173/full/. Accessed July 18, 2018.

13. The 340B discount program, policy brief. Michael McCaughan, Health Affairs; 2017. Available at: https://www.healthaffairs.org/do/10.1377/hpb20171024.663441/full/. Accessed July 18, 2018.

14. "CVS, aetna shares jump on report about deal's antitrust status," Zachary Tracer, Robert Langreth, Bloomberg News, Available at: https://www.bloomberg.com/news/articles/2018-07-12/cvs-aetna-shares-jump-on-report-about-deal-s-antitrust-status. Accessed July 18, 2018.

15. Thomas K, Abelson R, Bray C. Cigna to buy express scripts in $52 billion health care deal. New York Times 2018. Available at: https://www.nytimes.com/2018/03/08/business/dealbook/cigna-express-scripts.html. Accessed July 18, 2018.

Workforce Trends in Rheumatology

Adam Kilian, MD[a],*, Laura A. Upton, MD[b], Daniel F. Battafarano, DO[c],
Seetha U. Monrad, MD[a]

KEYWORDS

- Rheumatology • Workforce • Healthcare • Supply and demand
- Physician shortage • Utilization • Access to care

KEY POINTS

- The United States is facing a rheumatology provider shortage over the next decade, which will negatively affect care for patients with rheumatic disease across the nation if this deficit is not thoughtfully addressed.
- The increasing numbers of retiring rheumatology specialists, women entering the workforce, and rheumatology graduates seeking part-time employment were identified by the 2015 workforce study group as the most significant factors driving the projected decline in supply of providers.
- The major factors driving the projected increase in demand include an aging and growing population and improved treatment options, both of which increase disease prevalence and the challenge of managing chronic rheumatologic diseases.
- Innovative and multifaceted local, state, and federal strategies are necessary to provide adequate care for patients with rheumatic diseases.

INTRODUCTION

The United States is facing a critical physician shortage over the next decade, which could cause significant health care access issues for patients across the nation if this deficit is not thoughtfully addressed. The American Association of Medical College projects that physician demand will grow faster than supply, leading to a deficit of up to 120,000 physicians by 2030.[1] Much of the deficit between demand and supply is driven by population growth and aging.[1] Although the US population as a whole is projected to grow by nearly 11%, the population aged 65 years and older—which has the highest per capita consumption of health care of all age groups—is estimated to grow by 50%.[1] The aging population will also be associated

[a] Division of Rheumatology, Department of Internal Medicine, University of Michigan, 300 North Ingalls Building, Ann Arbor, Michigan 48109, USA; [b] Georgetown University, School of Medicine, Washington, DC, USA; [c] Department of Medicine, San Antonio Military Medical Center, 3551 Roger Brooke Drive, Fort Sam Houston, Texas 78234, USA
* Corresponding author. 1156 Concord Court, Northville, MI 48167.
E-mail address: adkilian@med.umich.edu

Rheum Dis Clin N Am 45 (2019) 13–26
https://doi.org/10.1016/j.rdc.2018.09.002
0889-857X/19/Published by Elsevier Inc.

rheumatic.theclinics.com

with a reduction of physician supply, since one-third of currently practicing physicians will surpass 65 years of age in the upcoming decade and many will retire or work part-time.[1] This physician shortage is expected to affect all medical specialties, including rheumatology. This article aims to (1) describe the evolution of the approaches to rheumatology workforce studies and modeling, (2) summarize our understanding of the current and projected US rheumatology workforce, and (3) discuss strategies to improve access to care for patients with rheumatic diseases.

HISTORY OF RHEUMATOLOGY WORKFORCE STUDIES

Since the 1990s, the American College of Rheumatology (ACR) has been conducting workforce studies that project the future capacity of the nation's rheumatology workforce. These studies have provided important information to help guide interventions from academic, public, and private sectors to meet the demands of the population and ensure delivery of high-quality and cost-efficient care to patients with rheumatologic conditions. The rapid pace of change in health care since the 1990s has required periodic reassessment to update the workforce projections and improve workforce study models.

Pre-2000 Workforce Studies

In 1980, the Graduate Medical Education National Advisory Committee (GMENAC) applied a needs-based model to estimate medical care requirements and physician supply for all medical and surgical specialties. The GMENAC study predicted a surplus of rheumatologists, estimating that by 1990 there would be 3000 rheumatologists in the United States, yet only 1900 would be needed to meet the estimated requirements for rheumatologic care.[2]

In 1990, the ACR commissioned an expert panel to revise the GMENAC requirements model by incorporating estimates of comorbidity prevalence, numbers of visits per patient with a particular rheumatic disease, and the proportion of visits that could be delegated to primary care providers (PCPs) or would not result in ongoing rheumatologic care. Estimated changes in population and disease prevalence were incorporated for future projections. This study concluded that there were approximately 3000 rheumatologists in the United States as of 1990, as predicted by the GMENAC study, representing a rheumatologist to population ratio of approximately 1:85,000. The revised needs-based model, however, concluded that the demand for rheumatologists (approximately 6000 rheumatologists required) substantially exceeded the supply, and projected that this supply-demand mismatch would worsen in upcoming decades (8100 rheumatologists required by 2010, yet only 4800 would be available).[2] This projection came at the time of a trend in which the number of internal medicine training program graduates entering rheumatology fellowships was decreasing. The study provided recommendations for narrowing the gap, such as increasing the number of training positions, enhancing recruitment efforts, and educating other physicians about the importance of rheumatology.[2]

The Health Security Act (1993) facilitated the development of integrated managed care networks that were expected to increase comprehensive coverage for Americans and offset predicted shortages of subspecialists.[3] A 1996 workforce study that was submitted to the ACR but not published incorporated expected increases in health maintenance organizations and management of rheumatic diseases by more PCPs and actually predicted a surplus of rheumatologists by 2000.[4] These expected increases and predictions, however, never materialized.[4]

2005 Workforce Study

In 2005 the ACR commissioned a new workforce study that updated the previous model by incorporating clinical productivity factors based on sex and age.[4,5] The study concluded that demand for adult rheumatologists would continue to outpace supply, projecting a dramatic increase for adult rheumatology services of 46% by 2025; yet supply of rheumatologists was predicted to increase by only 1.2% in the same period.[5] The demand was anticipated to exceed the supply by more than 2500 rheumatologists by 2025.[5] The major factors producing this excess demand were attributed to population growth; increases in the elderly population, which has a disproportionately high number of musculoskeletal disorders relative to other age groups; increases in per capita income; development of new technology and medical treatments; and an aging rheumatology workforce with a large proportion of baby boomers who were nearing retirement.[5] The study predicted that the rate of entry into rheumatology was approximately 143 per year, whereas the retirement rate of active rheumatologists was approximately 200 per year.[5]

In response to the projected need described in the 2005 workforce study, there was an increase in adult fellowship programs (108–113) and fellowship positions (398–468).[6] In addition, the Association of Rheumatology Health Professionals (ARHP) expanded educational opportunities including ACR online programs for nurse practitioners and physician assistants interested in rheumatology.[4,7,8]

THE 2015 RHEUMATOLOGY WORKFORCE STUDY

In 2015, acknowledging the dramatic changes in the health care and educational landscapes, the ACR commissioned the most recent workforce study.[9] To provide a more accurate understanding of access-to-care issues, this study adopted a patient-centered integrative approach to workforce modeling that built on the previous model by incorporating socioeconomic factors, access-to-care issues, and perceptions of need from patients themselves. To better understand the clinical productivity of the workforce, the 2015 study estimated the clinical full-time effort (FTE) in addition to the actual number of practitioners entering the workforce. For example, if a rheumatology practitioner provided clinical care only 50% of the work week, then their estimated clinical FTE would be 0.5. This overall estimation incorporated changing demographics and practice trends, such as a shift to a more female-predominant workforce, more anticipated part-time clinicians, increasing retirement rates, and changing practice patterns of younger physicians. Additional factors related to clinical productivity (such as proportion of practitioners in academic vs nonacademic settings and increasing numbers of international medical graduates [IMGs]) were also incorporated into the modeling. The workforce study provided projections on the supply of and demand for rheumatology services for the United States from 2015 through 2030.

Methods

Retrospective data was collected from multiple primary and secondary sources to strengthen assumptions for the integrated model.[9,10] Primary sources included surveys of ACR/ARHP members, current rheumatology fellows in training (FITs), and a cohort of rheumatology patients identified by the Arthritis Foundation. Secondary sources included the American Medical Association, American Board of Internal Medicine, American Board of Pediatrics, Rheumatology Nurses Society, and National Commission Certification of Physician Assistants, as well as data collected through focus groups interviews, and other published sources since 2005.[9,10]

Factors influencing supply included current rheumatology providers and associated demographic characteristics, succession planning and workload trends (eg, retirement, reduction in patient workload), practice patterns (eg, part-time vs full-time, FTEs), practice setting (nonacademic vs academic health center), number of new graduates entering the workforce, geographic distribution trends, and wage elasticities.[10] Factors influencing demand included health care utilization; disease prevalence across various demographic groups; changes in the population demographics, per capita income, and cost of rheumatology care; and access to care variables (physician per population and geographic trends).[10] The modeling did not assume equilibrium between supply and demand at baseline.

CURRENT CLINICAL RHEUMATOLOGY WORKFORCE

It is important to highlight that, because there is no single source for all US rheumatology demographic information, the baseline numbers of the active rheumatology workforce are in fact estimates that were based on the most reliable available data in 2015. Similarly, information regarding current practitioners and FITs varies depending on which source is used. We have attempted to clarify the source of data as much as possible.

Baseline Adult Rheumatology Workforce

The overall total number of active adult rheumatology providers in the United States in 2015—defined as rheumatologists, nurse practitioners (NPs), and physician assistants (PAs)—was estimated to be 6050 (clinical FTE of 5415): 5595 rheumatologists (FTE 4997), 248 NPs (FTE 228), and 207 PAs (FTE 190).[9,10] The estimation of adult rheumatologist FTEs represents an average of approximately 52,000 adults per adult rheumatologist in the United States.[10] Of the estimated total rheumatologists, 41% was identified as women and 59% as men[11]and nearly 75% identified as white.[10] In 2015, there was an estimated shortage of total clinical FTEs, with demand exceeding supply by approximately 700 clinical FTE (12.9%).

Baseline Pediatric Rheumatology Workforce

The overall total number of active pediatric rheumatology providers in the United States in 2015 was estimated to be 326 (clinical FTE of 311): 300 pediatric rheumatologists (FTE 287), 22 NPs (FTE 20), and 4 PAs (FTE 4).[10] The estimation of pediatric rheumatologist FTEs represents an average of approximately 261,000 children per pediatric rheumatologist in the United States.[10] Of the estimated total pediatric rheumatologists, 68% was identified as women and 32% as men and a large majority identified as white (**Table 1**).[10]

Practice Settings

Based on the available data, approximately 80% of adult rheumatologists worked in nonacademic settings, whereas approximately 20% worked in academic settings.[10] Nonacademic practitioners were found to work slightly fewer hours per week than academic practitioners yet would see more than twice as many patients each week.[10,12] In contrast, only 5% of pediatric rheumatologists work in nonacademic settings, with the vast majority practicing in academics.[10,13]

Geographic Distribution

Adult and pediatric rheumatologists in 2015 were found to be geographically maldistributed across the United States. The highest concentrations of adult rheumatologists

Table 1
2015 Adult and pediatric rheumatology workforce (ACR 2015)

Specialty Training	Adult		Pediatric	
	Total Numbers	Estimated Clinical FTE	Total Numbers	Estimated Clinical FTE
Rheumatologists	5595	4997	300	287
Nurse Practitioners	248	228	22	20
Physician Assistants	207	190	4	4
Total Active Primary Providers	6050	5415	326	311

From ACR Workforce Study Group (WSG). American College of Rheumatology. 2015 Workforce Study of Rheumatology Specialists in the United States. 2016. Available at: https://www.rheumatology.org/Learning-Center/Statistics/Workforce-Study.

were in the Northeast (21% of adult rheumatologists, 3.07 rheumatologists per 100,000 adults). The Mid-Atlantic, Great Lakes, and West regions all exceeded 2 rheumatologists per 100,000 adults and correlated with many major metropolitan areas in the United States. The lowest concentrations of adult rheumatologists occurred in the South Central, Southeast, and Southwest regions that had substantially lower ratios of 1.52, 1.41, and 1.28 rheumatologists per 100,000 adults, respectively.[10] The highest concentrations of pediatric rheumatologists were also in the Northeast (25% of pediatric rheumatologists, 0.83 rheumatologists per 100,000 children). The Mid-Atlantic, North Central, Northwest, and West regions all exceeded 0.5 rheumatologists per 100,000 children. The lowest concentrations of pediatric rheumatologists occurred in the Southwest, South Central, and Southeast regions that had substantially lower ratios of 0.17, 0.20, and 0.21 rheumatologists per 100,000 children, respectively.[10]

Rheumatology Fellows

In 2015, there were 497 adult and pediatric FITs distributed among 113 adult and 34 pediatric rheumatology programs in the United States. Most were women (57%), over half (53%) were IMGs, more than 75% had student loan debt greater than $100,000, and residency was the most common time they felt inspired to pursue rheumatology.[6,10] The most common reasons for pursuing rheumatology included intellectual interest, lifestyle/work hours, and clinical rotations. Private practice was the most commonly preferred career path overall.[14] Women reported more interest than men in pursuing a clinician educator track.[14] After fellowship, 11% of FITs reported planning to work part-time, which was more common for women than men, and 17.5% of FITs reported planning to practice outside the United States, the majority IMGs.[10,14]

PATIENT PERSPECTIVE

Adult patients, young adult patients, and parents of pediatric patients with rheumatic disease were surveyed as part of the 2015 workforce study to help inform access to care issues. Approximately 48% of adult, 40% of young adult, and 55% of pediatric patients were diagnosed by a rheumatologist, with the remainder diagnosed by their PCP or a nonrheumatology specialist.[15] Thirty percent of adults and 26% of young adult and pediatric patients had over a 4-month wait to see a rheumatologist after the onset of their symptoms.[15] There was a large difference in the ease of making routine follow-up appointments within the recommended time frame between adult and pediatric patients; 78% of adult patients reported they were able to do so, compared with only 57% of pediatric and young adult patients.[15] More than half of all patients indicated it was very difficult to make urgent care appointments with their rheumatologist and often relied on their PCP for urgent care when they could not see their rheumatologist.[15] Approximately half of survey respondents (53% of adult, 46% of pediatric and young adult patients) had access to a rheumatologist less than 2 hours from their home. Patients reported significant indirect costs associated with their rheumatology care, including fuel, overnight lodging, missing work to get to appointments, and child care.[10]

PROJECTED WORKFORCE

The projected demand for adult and pediatric rheumatology services greatly outpaces the projected supply of the rheumatology workforce. Supply and demand projections from the 2015 workforce study portend a dramatic decline in the adult and pediatric rheumatology workforce from 2015 to 2030. This projected decline is greater than that was projected in the 2005 workforce study.[4]

Adult Rheumatology Providers

Supply: it is projected that there will be a decline in supply of adult rheumatology provider clinical FTEs: 5027 by 2020 (−7.8% from 2015), 4221 by 2025 (−22.6% from 2015), and 3974 by 2030 (−27.1% from 2015).[10]

Demand: over the same period, it is projected that there will be an increase in the demand of adult rheumatology clinical FTEs: 6796 by 2020 (+36% from 2015), 7490 by 2025 (+49.9% from 2015), and 8184 by 2030 (+63.8% from 2015).[10]

Shortage: the projected shortage of total adult rheumatology clinical FTEs is therefore estimated at 1769 by 2020 (35% of estimated active workforce), 3269 by 2025 (78% of estimated active workforce), and 4210 by 2030 (106% of estimated active workforce).

Pediatric Rheumatology Providers

Supply: it is projected that there will be a decline in supply of pediatric rheumatology provider clinical FTEs: 291 by 2020 (−7% from 2015), 272 by 2025 (−13.1% from 2015), and 261 by 2030 (−16.6% from 2015).[16]

Demand: over the same period, it is projected that there will be an increase in the demand of pediatric rheumatology clinical FTEs: 407 by 2020 (+41.8% from 2015), 434 by 2025 (+51.2% from 2015), and 461 by 2030 (+60.6% from 2015).[10]

Shortage: the projected shortage of total adult rheumatology clinical FTEs is therefore estimated at 116 by 2020 (40% of estimated active workforce), 162 by 2025 (60% of estimated active workforce), and 200 by 2030 (77% of estimated active workforce) (**Fig. 1**).

KEY FACTORS AFFECTING THE SUPPLY AND DEMAND OF RHEUMATOLOGY PROVIDERS

Multiple factors are expected to contribute to the worsening supply and demand mismatch of adult rheumatology providers. The increasing numbers of retiring rheumatology specialists and rheumatology graduates seeking part-time employment (including higher numbers of women) were identified by the 2015 workforce study group as the most significant factors driving the projected decline in supply of FTE. The major factors driving the projected increase in demand include an aging and growing population and improved treatment options, both of which increase disease

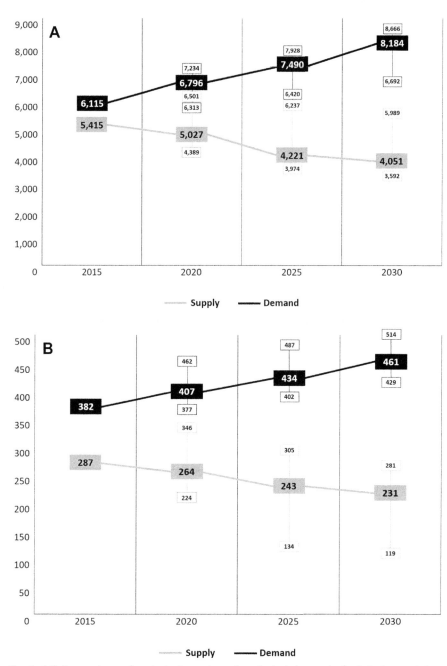

Fig. 1. (A) Comparison of projected supply and projected demand of adult rheumatology providers (clinical FTEs) along with best- and worst-case scenario projections, 2015 to 2030; includes NPs and PAs in the totals. (B) Comparison of projected supply and projected demand of pediatric rheumatology providers (clinical FTEs) along with best- and worst-case scenario projections, 2015 to 2030; because of lack of availability data, NPs and PAs are not included in the totals. (*Adapted from* [A] Battafarano DF, Ditmyer M, Bolster MB, et al. 2015 American College of Rheumatology workforce study: supply and demand projections of

prevalence and the challenge of managing chronic rheumatologic diseases. Here, the authors provide a summary of the major contributing factors.

Supply Factors

Current rheumatology workforce
In 2015, there was already an estimated shortage of total adult and pediatric rheumatology clinical FTEs, with demand exceeding supply by approximately 700 clinical FTEs (13%) for adults and 95 clinical FTEs (25%) for children.[10,17]

Number of new graduates entering the workforce
The number of available fellowship positions, the fill-rate of those positions, graduation rates, and number of IMGs who anticipate remaining in the United States were assumed to remain constant in the supply model.[10] Workforce projections indicate a gender shift in the rheumatology workforce with more women than men expected to enter the rheumatology workforce each year: this trend is significant when considering clinical FTEs because historically women are more likely than men to work part-time. Overall, graduating fellows who enter the workforce from 2015 to 2030 are projected to more likely seek part-time employment.

Succession planning trends
The rate at which rheumatologists leave practice represents another factor that affects the supply of rheumatologists. The rheumatology workforce is aging, with a large portion of baby boomers (51% in 2015) who are reaching retirement; in fact, half of adult rheumatologists plan to retire within the next 10 years.[10] There are many reasons provided for why rheumatologists are leaving or planning to leave the workforce, including retirement, mortality, disability, and changes in career patterns.[10] The workforce study survey indicated that approximately 50% of adult and 32% of pediatric/Med-Ped rheumatologists and 43% of midlevel practitioners plan to retire within the next 10 years.[10]

Workload trends
Physician workload is often measured in terms of total patient care hours worked or number of patients seen within a given period of time. The 2015 workforce study identified a significant decrease in the average number of annual patient visits for rheumatology providers compared with 2005, with an overall average decrease in patient load per week of about 19% for women and 14% for men.[10] This decrease has been attributed to several provider practice trends that are predicted to continue. Many baby boomers who compose the rheumatology workforce are nearing retirement and plan to decrease their patient load: in fact, approximately 60% of nonacademic practitioners and 40% of academicians plan to reduce their patient load in the next 10 years by up to 50%.[12] Millennials generally place more emphasis on the value of work-life balance than the baby boomers, and so as rheumatology graduates continue entering the workforce they are more likely to seek part-time employment and/or treat fewer patients per year than rheumatology practitioners of past years. Furthermore, the anticipated percentage of women entering the rheumatology workforce is expected to surpass the percentage of men by

---

adult rheumatology workforce, 2015–2030. Arthritis Care Res (Hoboken) 2018;70(4):623, with permission; and [B] Battafarano DF. 2015 workforce study of rheumatology specialists in the United States: 2016 pediatric rheumatology workforce. 2016 ACR/ARHP Annual Meeting. Washington, DC, September 28, 2016, with permission.)

2020: based on survey responses and published literature, this distribution change is projected to reduce working hours by 7 per week and annual patient visits by 30%.[9]

Practice inefficiencies greatly contribute to workload trends and affect provider satisfaction and retention. As part of the workforce study, rheumatologists identified the top 10 most common and pervasive barriers to practice: (1) insurance issues (eg, poor reimbursement, preauthorization, low contract), (2) Electronic Health Record implementation, (3) lack of staff, (4) incentives not aligned properly, (5) Physician Quality Reporting System too bothersome, (6) poor administrative support, (7) lack of loan repayment options, (8) high-cost medications for patients, (9) difficult recruiting, and (10) lack of time with patients.[12]

Geographic distribution trends

The geographic maldistribution of rheumatologists across the United States is predicted to worsen over the next 15 years. By 2025, the most US regions will have less than 1 rheumatologist per 100,000 adults. The Northwest is expected to be the most affected, with an anticipated decrease to 0.50 rheumatologists per 100,000 adults (**Fig. 2**, **Table 2**).

Demand Factors

Health care utilization trends

Rapidly expanding treatment options for rheumatologic diseases, such as novel biological and oral synthetic disease-modifying antirheumatic drugs, increase the need for patient access to health care professionals.[18] Furthermore, novel treatment strategies for rheumatologic diseases such as treat-to-target, in which composite measures of disease activity are used to adapt therapy for each individual patient, increase the need for time spent with a health care professional.

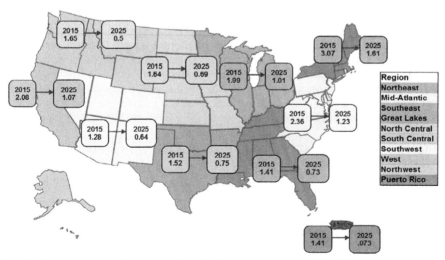

Fig. 2. Adult rheumatology provider distribution rate per 100,000 patients in 2015 compared with projections for 2025. (*From* Battafarano DF, Ditmyer M, Bolster MB, et al. 2015 American College of Rheumatology workforce study: supply and demand projections of adult rheumatology workforce, 2015–2030. Arthritis Care Res (Hoboken) 2018;70(4):621; with permission.)

Table 2
Population projections for pediatric rheumatology in United States

	Baseline	2020	2025	2030
Number projected with disease	300,000	461,936	475,406	505,099
Children with disease/physician (supply)	1045.3	1974.1	3547.8	4244.5
Children with disease/physician (need)	681.8	999.9	976.2	982.7

Data from Battafarano DF. 2015 workforce study of rheumatology specialists in the united states: 2016 pediatric rheumatology workforce. 2016 ACR/ARHP Annual Meeting, Washington, DC. September 28, 2016.

Prevalence of disease and changes in population demographics

As the US population ages, the prevalence of doctor-diagnosed arthritis is expected to increase. By 2030, approximately 70 million Americans are predicted to be at risk for developing osteoarthritis, and although there is limited data informing the percentage of osteoarthritis patients that rheumatologists treat regularly (estimated as 25% in the 2015 ACR workforce study),[9] this large population of patients with osteoarthritis is expected to increase demand for rheumatologic services. As diagnostic and therapeutic strategies continue to improve, the prevalence of many rheumatologic conditions is expected to increase, further increasing demand for rheumatologic services. The prevalence of rheumatoid arthritis has already been shown to be on the rise, especially among aging women.[19] The number of children with rheumatologic disease is also projected to increase, from a baseline of approximately 300,000 in 2015 to more than 500,000 by 2030.

Per capita income

Based on per capita income compound growth from 2010 to 2015 and the forecasted value for 2020, an estimated compound growth for 2015 to 2025 will be approximately 2.5%, which is up 1.5% from 2005.[10] As the average household income increases, utilization of rheumatologic services is expected to increase as well.

Access to care variables

Many proposed changes in health policy aim to improve access to health care, such as increasing insurance coverage, funding initiatives that take care directly to target populations, and addressing social determinants of health. Improved health care access is expected to increase health care utilization as well, thus increasing demand, especially among communities with vulnerable patient populations who may benefit the most from health policy initiatives.

STRATEGIES TO ENSURE ACCESS TO CARE FOR PATIENTS WITH RHEUMATIC DISEASE

These projections are in parallel with the projections for a national physician shortage and shortages in other subspecialities.[1,9] Addressing the gap between supply and demand requires a multifaceted approach to ensure effective rheumatologic care for the US population. Here, the authors provide a summary of potential strategies that may be considered to address challenges that face the rheumatology workforce.

Innovate Medical Education

Both earlier and expanded exposure to musculoskeletal medicine and rheumatology for health students (MD, DO, PA, NP) and residents (pediatric and internal medicine) may stimulate more interest in rheumatology among trainees and enhance recruitment of providers into the field.[10,20] There are some indications that this is already occurring.[20]

Expand Fellowship Training

Increasing fellowship positions in underserved areas may help correct disparities in regional distribution of rheumatologists.[10] Providing rheumatology fellowships for allied health providers that focus on the most prevalent rheumatologic diseases (ie, gout, rheumatoid arthritis, spondyloarthropathies, Sjogren syndrome, polymyalgia rheumatica, juvenile arthritis) as well as osteoarthritis and fibromyalgia may help address some of the anticipated workforce gap.

Retain Rheumatology Providers

Retention strategies for IMGs who are completing US training to stay in the United States and aging rheumatology providers with plans for early retirement to retain part-time practice (10–30 hours per week) should be explored.

Improve Competencies in Rheumatology for Primary Care Providers

Guidelines for rheumatology consultation as well as integrating fundamental musculoskeletal and rheumatology curricula into primary care residencies may reduce primary care delays in recognizing early rheumatic diseases, improve timely rheumatology consultation, reduce unnecessary referrals, and facilitate direct referral to physical therapists and occupational therapists for primary musculoskeletal diagnoses.[9,21,22]

Empower Patients

Improving knowledge delivery to patients about their rheumatologic diseases and therapies has the potential to enhance their autonomy, quality of life, and ability to recognize and control early disease exacerbations. This may be accomplished by improving point-of-care teaching aids, tailoring self-study resources to patients' ages, health literacies, and computer access (online Websites and videos, magazines, brochures, handouts), as well as providing dedicated clinic visits (individual or for patient groups) for education by a midlevel practitioner or trainee. Policy changes to provide reimbursement for patient education may facilitate these enhancements to patient care. Easy-to-use handouts and smartphone apps may facilitate self-monitoring of disease activity. Disease-specific reference cards may be given to patients to assist nonrheumatologic providers should the patient require urgent or emergent care.

Improve Practice Efficiency

Disseminating practice efficiency strategies, building rheumatology-specific tools in the electronic health record, and maximizing the potential of midlevel practitioners to assist with chronic care patients may improve clinic productivity and provider retention. Patients could also monitor and submit treat-to-target goals electronically to rheumatology nurses or providers.

Increase Reimbursement

Implementation of alternative payment models that improve the way cognitive work is valued in evaluation and management codes—so that reimbursements reflect the value of care provided by cognitive (nonprocedural) specialists—may help focus care for patients who require it the most, attract more trainees to the field of rheumatology, and help support the existing and future workforce.[23]

Correct Regional Disparities

Financial incentive programs that offer scholarships or loan repayment/forgiveness may attract rheumatology providers to underserved communities where access to care is limited.[24–26] Increasing fellowship positions in underserved areas may also help correct the maldistribution of rheumatologists by local retention in close proximity to training.[6,10]

Improve Telemedicine Technology and Expand Telerheumatology Programs

Telerheumatology should include (1) digital screening of consultations to identify early rheumatic diseases and minimize consultations for nonrheumatology problems and (2) asynchronous electronic consultations providing rheumatology guidance and (3) synchronous video consultations from more remote sites to assist PCPs. Video synchronous telemedicine can be a potentially suitable modality for screening/triaging patient referrals and close monitoring of patients at high risk for disease flares and/or hospitalizations who have an established diagnosis. More research is required to confirm the validity and reliability of telerheumatology methods.[27,28]

Health Policy Reform

Any legislation that curtails insurance barriers, improves reimbursements for cognitive care services, increases funding for underserved communities, improves access to care for patients, and facilitates other creative solutions to offset the projected shortage of rheumatology services has the potential for state and federal health system improvement.

SUMMARY

The United States is facing a rheumatology provider shortage over the next decade, which will negatively affect care for patients with rheumatic disease across the nation if this deficit is not thoughtfully addressed. Over the next decade, the combination of an aging patient population, baby boomer retirements, changing demographics of incoming providers, imbalanced geographic distribution of rheumatology providers, and evolving health policies will significantly affect rheumatologic health care. It is estimated that by 2030, demand for rheumatology providers will be twice the available supply. Innovative and multifaceted local, state, and federal strategies are necessary to provide adequate care for patients with rheumatic diseases.

REFERENCES

1. American Association of Medical Colleges. 2018 update; the complexities of physician supply and demand: Projections from 2016 to 2030. Washinton, DC 2018.
2. Marder WD, Meenan RF, Felson DT, et al. The present and future adequacy of rheumatology manpower. A study of health care needs and physician supply. Arthritis Rheum 1991;34(10):1209–17. Available at: https://www.ncbi.nlm.nih.gov/pubmed/1930309.
3. Weiner JP. Forecasting the effects of health reform on US physician workforce requirement. evidence from HMO staffing patterns. JAMA 1994;272(3):222–30. Accessed Jul 2, 2018.
4. Deal CL, Hooker R, Harrington T, et al. The united states rheumatology workforce: Supply and demand, 2005-2025. Arthritis Rheum 2007;56(3):722–9. Available at: http://www.ncbi.nlm.nih.gov/pubmed/17328042.

5. Hogan PF, Bouchery E, for the American College of Rheumatology. 2005 work-force study of rheumatologists: Final report. 2006. Available at: https://www.rheumatology.org/Portals/0/Files/LewinReport.pdf. Accessed July 2, 2018.
6. Bolster MB, Bass AR, Hausmann JS, et al. 2015 rheumatology workforce study. The role of graduate medical education in adult rheumatology. Arthritis Rheumatol 2018;70(6):817–25.
7. Accreditation Council for Graduate Medical Education. Data resource book. Academic year 2014–2015. 2016. Available at: https://www.acgme-i.org/Portals/0/Databook/2014-2015_ACGMEInternational_Databook.pdf. Accessed July 2, 2018.
8. National Resident Matching Program. Results and data: 2015 main residency match. 2015. https://URL: http://www. nrmp.org/wp-content/uploads/2015/05/Main-Match-Results-and-Data-2015_final.pdf. Accessed July 2, 2018.
9. Battafarano DF, Ditmyer M, Bolster MB, et al. 2015 American college of rheumatology workforce study: Supply and demand projections of adult rheumatology workforce, 2015–2030. Arthritis Care Res 2018;70(4):617–26.
10. American College of Rheumatology. 2015 workforce study of rheumatology specialists in the United States Atlanta, GA. 2016.
11. Deal C, Bolster MB, Hausmann JS, et al. 2015 ACR/ARHP Workforce Study (WFS): Adult Rheumatology Specialists in the United States: Effect of Gender and Generation [abstract number 89]. *Arthritis Rheumatol* 2016;68(suppl 10).
12. Monrad S, Battafarano D, Ditmyer M. Academic and Non-Academic Rheumatology: Practice Trends and Common Barriers to Practice from the 2015 ACR/ARHP Workforce Study Survey [abstract number 99]. *Arthritis Rheumatol* 2016; 68(suppl 10).
13. Battafarano D, Monrad S, Ditmyer M, et al. 2015 ACR/ARHP Workforce Study in the United States: Pediatric Rheumatologist Supply and Demand Projections for 2015-2030 [abstract number 927]. *Arthritis Rheumatol* 2016;68(suppl 10).
14. Hausmann JS, Monrad S, Ditmyer M, et al. The Future of Rheumatology: Pediatric and Adult Fellows-in-Training Results from the 2015 ACR/ARHP Workforce Study [abstract number 1140]. *Arthritis Rheumatol* 2016;68(suppl 10).
15. Monrad S, Imundo L, Battafarano D, Ditmyer M. Access to Care: The Patient Perspective from the 2015 ACR/ARHP Workforce Study [abstract number 1248]. *Arthritis Rheumatol* 2016;68(suppl 10).
16. Gupta S, Black-Schaffer WS, Crawford JM, et al. An innovative interactive modeling tool to analyze scenario-based physician workforce supply and demand. Acad Pathol 2015;2(4). 237428951560673.
17. Battafarano DF. 2015 workforce study of rheumatology specialists in the united states: 2016 pediatric rheumatology workforce. Washinton, DC: 2016 ACR/ARHP Annual Meeting. September 28, 2016.
18. Solomon DH, Bitton A, Fraenkel L, et al. Roles of nurse practitioners and physician assistants in rheumatology practices in the US. Arthritis Care Res 2014; 66(7):1108–13.
19. Myasoedova E, Crowson CS, Kremers HM, et al. Is the incidence of rheumatoid arthritis rising?: Results from olmsted county, minnesota, 1955-2007. Arthritis Rheum 2010;62(6):1576–82. Available at: https://www.ncbi.nlm.nih.gov/pubmed/20191579.
20. Tran HW, Mathias LM, Panush RS. Has rheumatology become a more attractive career choice? Comparison of trends in the rheumatology fellowship match from 2008 to 2013 with 2014 to 2017. Arthritis Care Res 2018. https://doi.org/10.1002/acr.23691. Available at: https://www.ncbi.nlm.nih.gov/pubmed/29953744.

21. Riley L, Harris C, McKay M, et al. The role of nurse practitioners in delivering rheumatology care and services: results of a U.S. survey. J Am Assoc Nurse Pract 2017;29(11):673–81.
22. Bykerk V, Emery P. Delay in receiving rheumatology care leads to long-term harm. Arthritis Rheum 2010;62(12):3519–21.
23. American College of Rheumatology. 2018 ACR health policy statements. Atlanta, GA; 2018.
24. Opoku ST, Apenteng BA, Lin G, et al. A comparison of the J-1 visa waiver and loan repayment programs in the recruitment and retention of physicians in rural nebraska. J Rural Health 2015;31(3):300–9.
25. Grobler L, Marais BJ, Mabunda S. Interventions for increasing the proportion of health professionals practicing in rural and other underserved areas. Cochrane Database Syst Rev 2015;(6). CD005314. https://www.ncbi.nlm.nih.gov/pubmed/26123126.
26. Tierney J, Terhune K. Expanding the national health service corps scholarship program to general surgery: a proposal to address the national shortage of general surgeons in the united states. JAMA Surg 2017;152(4):315–6.
27. Ward IM, Schmidt TW, Lappan C, et al. How critical is tele-medicine to the rheumatology workforce? Arthritis Care Res 2016;68(10):1387–9.
28. McDougall JA, Ferucci ED, Glover J, et al. Telerheumatology: a systematic review. Arthritis Care Res 2017;69(10):1546–57.

Challenges to Practicing Rheumatology in an Academic Center

Sobia Hassan, MD, MRCP[a], Meghan M. Smith, MHA[b],
Joel A. Block, MD[b], Meenakshi Jolly, MD[c],*

KEYWORDS

- Challenges • Academics • Rheumatology • Mentorship • Research • Teaching
- Clinical care

KEY POINTS

- There are challenges associated with all aspects of academic rheumatology, including patient care, education, research, and professional development.
- Greater emphasis on the generation of revenue from clinical activities has meant less time and resources for academic pursuits.
- Collaboration between academic institutions, professional societies, and federal institutions is required to come up with viable solutions for these challenges.

INTRODUCTION

There are myriad advantages associated with practicing rheumatology in an academic setting: intellectual stimulation, choice of varied career tracks (**Table 1**), access to multidisciplinary specialists and state of the art technology, and the security of a guaranteed salary and benefits.

There also many challenges, however, and these are the focus of this article. A review of previously published work on this topic reveals a paucity of rheumatology-specific literature; so in formulating this article, work addressing the challenges faced by the authors' colleagues in other medical specialties is also cited. Additionally, much of this article is based on the experiences and opinions of the authors and colleagues at various academic centers. This article (1) considers the challenges of maintaining an adequate academic workforce in the coming decades; (2) discusses issues involved in

Disclosures: None relevant to this work.
[a] Division of Rheumatology, Rush University Medical Center, 1611 West Harrison Street Suite 510, Chicago, IL 60612, USA; [b] Division of Rheumatology, Department of Medicine, Rush University Medical Center, 1611 West Harrison Street Suite 510, Chicago, IL 60612, USA; [c] Division of Rheumatology, Rush University Medical Center, 1611 West Harrison Street Suite 510, Chicago, IL 60612, USA
* Corresponding author.
E-mail address: Meenakshi_Jolly@rush.edu

Rheum Dis Clin N Am 45 (2019) 27–37
https://doi.org/10.1016/j.rdc.2018.09.003
rheumatic.theclinics.com

Table 1 Various academic tracks and their descriptions	
Academic Track	**Description**
Investigator	100% effort devoted to research
Clinical investigator	Majority of effort in research, with a balance in clinical care
Clinician educator	Majority of effort in clinical care with a portion devoted to education
Clinician-educator-administrator	Majority of effort in clinical care with a portion devoted to education and administration
Clinician-education-scholar	Majority of effort in clinical care, with a balance in education and expected to engage in scholarly activities
Clinician scholar	Majority of effort in clinical care but expected to engage in scholarly activities
Clinician	100% Effort devoted to clinical care; still expected to play a role in education, especially in clinical care setting

each of the various aspects of academic rheumatology: education, research, and clinical care; and (3) discusses issues in health care management and professional development.

CONCERNS FOR WORKFORCE SHORTAGES

An important challenge that the entire field of rheumatology faces is the expected shortage of rheumatologists in the near future. Projections derived from data obtained from the 2015 American College of Rheumatology (ACR) Workforce Study estimate that there will be a 25% decrease in supply of clinical providers in 2030 compared with 2015 levels and that demand will exceed supply by 102%.[1] There are many reasons for this supply and demand imbalance, including (1) attrition of rheumatologists due to baby boomer retirements and an increase in part-time providers; (2) the aging of the US population, with an estimated 25% of the projected adult population having doctor-diagnosed arthritis in 2030 (67 million compared with 52 million in 2012)[2]; and (3) maldistribution of the workforce because a majority of rheumatologists tend to favor working in metropolitan areas, in the vicinity of their place of training, leaving the rural population especially neglected.[1]

Future workforce shortages will be especially detrimental to academic institutions that are already struggling to maintain their limited workforce. Although the exact distribution of the rheumatology workforce is unknown, it is estimated that only 20% of rheumatologists work in the academic setting and increasing numbers of junior academic rheumatologists are transitioning into nonacademic positions than ever before due to difficulty with academic advancement and tenure, insecure research funding, higher salary opportunities, and student loan debt.[3]

In efforts to attract more physicians to academics, the factors that influence career choice need to be understood. Those wishing to pursue a career in academic medicine are driven by a desire to teach, conduct research, and provide care to a complex and challenging set of patients in an environment of intellectual stimulation.[4] Participation in research during medical school and residency and the influence of a mentor in academic medicine have been identified as factors associated with a career in academic medicine, and trainees' interest in academic medicine decreases as they progress through their residency.[4]

Lower pay and lack of autonomy are factors that discourage physicians from a career in academic medicine.[4] The salary of rheumatologists falls in the bottom third of all specialties, according to a 2018 Medscape Physician Compensation Report, and those in academics make less than their counterparts in private practice. With a majority of new doctors starting their career with a mean educational debt of $173,000, this becomes a major factor when choosing career path.[5]

To attract more physicians to academics, creative ways are needed that attract, retain and nurture academic rheumatologists starting from medical school.

SPECIFIC CHALLENGES BY MISSIONS OF ACADEMIC INSTITUTIONS
Education

> As a clinical educator at a large tertiary institution the biggest challenge has been finding time and justifying effort as a teacher and mentor. The core of this job entails professional and personal counseling on many levels. However, often the only surrogate to measure the success of these roles comes as the number of abstracts or publications. Education, mentee satisfaction, personal and professional growth, which often take significantly more effort, are hard to measure and are thus not accounted for. In addition, in a day and age of increasing clinical demands there is much less value placed on such roles.
> —Comments from a clinician educator at an academic institution.

A majority of those practicing in academic medicine have a role in educating students, residents, and fellows. Some have more formal roles as clinical educators or clinician-educator-administrators, where they have some percentage of their full-time equivalent devoted to teaching.

Those in academics are expected to teach in a variety of settings, such as at the bedside, during formal lectures, and at regional and national courses or conferences. Although junior faculty are expected to be efficient in all these aspects of teaching, they often have little experience or formal training in how to do so. It, therefore, would be beneficial to have faculty development programs that teach the skills necessary to be a successful educator.

A majority of clinical teaching takes place in the increasingly busy outpatient setting or during inpatient rounds and the challenge becomes how to balance patient care with teaching. The other challenge is how to remain clinically up to date so as to ensure a quality education for trainees. This is especially important given the speed with which new developments and other advances are occurring in rheumatology. Attending conferences and workshops to learn and become certified in new skills (such as ultrasound or bone densitometry) requires not only time but also financial resources. Additionally, the time needed to integrate these new skills into patient care and to teach these skills to trainees often translates into loss of clinical productivity.

Large numbers of teaching hospitals lack rheumatology training programs. Hence, academic institutions have been accommodating increasing numbers of outside rotators who come from programs without rheumatology exposure. This places increased pressure on academic faculty whose teaching efforts often go unsupported or remunerated because there are usually no educational contracts between the academic center and these community programs.

Although academic institutions are faced with greater patient volume and an anticipated shortage of rheumatologists, funding for fellowship training slots has not increased. To address these issues and combat trainee fatigue, additional funding to support additional fellowship training spots is much needed.

There are also a number of unique challenges faced by clinician educators and clinician-educator-administrators.

The path for promotion for clinician educators is less clearly defined at many academic centers, and a focus on teaching does not usually yield the grants and publications that are seen as the traditional requirements for promotion. Educational activities, such as lecturing at other institutions or professional societies, can provide evidence of regional or national recognition but are usually not supported financially by the lecturer's institution.

Finally, clinician-educator-administrators face additional time-intensive challenges dealing with the ever-evolving and complicated process of accreditation and compliance for the training program, while ensuring that trainees adhere to such requirements as the Accreditation Council for Graduate Medical Education milestone evaluation.

Research

Balancing clinical responsibilities and research endeavors, I believe is one of the greatest challenges for clinical investigators. One cannot just push patient care to the side just because a grant deadline is approaching. As a clinical investigator, my drive comes from the pursuit of knowledge and discovering something new for the first time. I could even say I enjoy writing papers and grants. I could do without the constant critiques which sometime seem more like an academic exercise by the reviewer than truly collaborative encouragement in the pursuit of knowledge. I could do without academic politics.

I have difficulties when planning my research because of the bureaucracy burden, so many rules that make everything time consuming and complicated. It would be of great value to have more supportive research personal and administrative personnel to help answer questions and prepare proposals. In summary, someone willing to facilitate the process instead of making everything more difficult. Other additional challenges are having enough time to mentor fellows and students with small research projects, and to submit grants and get external funding.
— Comments from clinical researchers at an academic center.

A study by Ogdie and colleagues[6] found that 23% of rheumatologists switched career path from research to another track a median of 7 years after completing fellowship. The factors associated with a successful transition to independent researcher, or failure to launch, were funding, institutional support, and mentorship. Other reasons cited for leaving research included clinical burden, insufficient protected time for research, financial struggles, other opportunities in administration or teaching, relocation to an area without research opportunities, need for job security, and fear of failure in funding or achieving tenure.[6]

More than 60% of researchers surveyed by Ogdie and colleagues[6] were women. Women in their reproductive years face additional challenges managing work-life balance with research and may struggle to meet the time-sensitive milestones required for promotion or tenure.[7]

Funding

Most researchers in academic institutes struggle to fund their research throughout their career, and obtaining funding remains one of the major hurdles cited in starting and maintaining a research career.[6] Due to financial stressors, academic institutions are often unwilling to support adequate protected time and to provide start-up packages that permit new investigators to complete preliminary studies from which to base competitive grant applications.[8]

Federal funding sources have declined since 2003, and there is stiff competition for both career development awards (K series) and later independent grants (R series) from the National Institutes of Health (NIH). In addition, the funding for research in the rheumatic diseases has always been substantially lower than that of other prevalent diseases, such as cardiovascular diseases or cancer. Funding from philanthropic sources has also dwindled or tends to be given to specialties like orthopedics where (1) the impact of what they do is more visible to the public, (2) the demographics of patients are more suited to philanthropic cause given their stage in life and availability of resources, and (3) they are on the institutions' preferred priority list as the top net revenue generators.[8] Rheumatologists need to do a better job in advertising the importance and impact of their research and discoveries to the community.

Additionally, many funding grants are only for short terms; thus, researchers are under pressure to complete all study processes within the stipulated time period, while also applying for more grants so they can avoid unfunded periods.[8]

Finally, even fully funded investigators do not generate sufficient resources through grants to cover all research-related costs, and increasingly restrictive federal policies have made it even more difficult to fund full salary and administrative support for senior clinical investigators. Directing some of the downstream revenue generated for the institution by its rheumatologists could help provide bridge funding for unfunded periods and provide protected time for early career investigators.

Writing grants

Most junior faculty do not know the nuances of grant submission and budget development and may not have the mentoring and infrastructure support required to help them. Grant writing for foundation, pharmaceutical, and philanthropic sources of funding each has its own specifications and templates, which can make the process frustrating and repetitive.

Grant writing is also competitive and young researchers may be at a disadvantage, because large funding agencies tend to favor more senior and established researchers. The average age of NIH R01 principal investigators was 51 for all investigators and 42 for first-time investigators in 2007.[9]

A majority of academic faculty have multiple failed grant applications. NIH data show that NIH R01 success rates fell from 26% in 2000 to 16.7% in 2017.[10] Once a grant attempt has failed, researchers may become discouraged and unwilling to pursue further attempts at grant submission or resubmission.

Where available, the help of mentors, grant writing workshops, and master's programs may be invaluable for researchers but these require institutional support, finances, and personal time commitment.

Clinical trials

Researchers involved in clinical trials face several challenges: (1) dealing with complex regulatory burdens required by trial sponsors and institutional review boards, (2) training and certification in the use of complex assessment tools (eg, British Isles Lupus Assessment Group (BILAG) or Systemic Lupus Erythematosus Disease Activity Index (SLEDAI)) not routinely used in clinical practice, (3) high-level data documentation requirements, (4) limited and often insufficient budgets, (5) the need to find other physicians willing to evaluate clinical trial patients when the principal investigator is unavailable, (6) time pressures associated with traveling to meetings and protocol training, and (7) difficulties meeting patient recruitment targets due to strict inclusion criteria, competition from other trials recruiting similar patients, and reservations among minority groups.[11]

Clinical Care

Provision of health care was and remains the main mission of most every academic institution.

Patient population

Many of the challenges are similar in academic vs non-academic multi-specialty group settings. Limits of decision making control are an issue in both settings. There are likely to be more socially disadvantaged patients as a challenge in many academic settings.

I am expected to perform at a superior level, often times seeing challenging patients who come for second or third opinion at times with mountains of records to be reviewed in the same time frame a community rheumatologist would see patients. I am also required to meet unrealistic productivity targets, all while teaching the new generation of trainees.
                 —*Comments from full-time clinicians at an academic institution.*

The patient population at academic medical centers tends to be more complex because they attract patients seeking second or third opinions or referrals from community rheumatologists struggling to deal with patients who have failed standard therapies or who pose a diagnostic dilemma. A considerable amount of time, often more than allotted for the visit, is spent on evaluating these complex patients and requesting and reviewing their records. Higher levels of complexity, time, and effort, however, do not always yield higher work relative value units (wRVUs.)

In addition, unlike private practice, academic centers may not have the option to screen out patients based on their insurance or other variables that may be associated with greater need for patient education and social support.

Electronic health records

One of the consequences of seeing a large number of patients is dealing with the ever-increasing documentation requirements of electronic medical records. There are multiple electronic health record (EHR) platforms, most of which do not cross-talk, and physicians working at different academic centers may have to learn the nuances of each system. Additionally, the commonly used EHR platforms are clearly more geared toward capturing billing and physician quality measures than toward clinical utility or end-user ease of use. In many academic institutions, physicians are faced with penalties for not closing charts in a timely manner or for delays in responding to patient messages and refill requests.

Time spent dealing with EHRs not only takes away from quality time spent with the patient but also adds to physician frustration. Results from the 2015 ACR Workforce Study showed that rheumatologists working in both academic and nonacademic settings identified dealing with EHRs as well as insurance issues as their top 2 barriers to practice.[12]

A study published in the *Annals of Internal Medicine* looking at the allocation of physician time in the ambulatory setting showed that only 27% of a physician's day is spent on direct clinical face time with patients, whereas 50% is spent on EHR documentation and desk work. Physicians also reported spending 1 hour to 2 hours on EHR work after work.[13]

Super-specializing and specialty clinics

There is an expectation that academic rheumatologists should subspecialize within their field and they are encouraged to set up disease-focused specialty clinics (eg, lupus, vasculitis, and myositis clinics). Although this allows physicians to stand out from their peers and develop research interests, it also puts them under additional pressure to find their niche. Faculty often struggle to learn the logistics of starting and running such subspecialty clinics with little guidance and limited resources.

Satellite clinics

In efforts to expand outreach, institutions are developing more community clinics and forming alliances with community hospitals. Physicians employed in these facilities deal with more credentialing and paperwork, spend more time traveling, and may be expected to partake in more clinical duties with less time for scholarly activities compared with their peers.

Challenges for the pure clinician

Most physicians joining new facilities are expected to start with 100% clinical effort, unless they come with extramural funding or have departmental support that protects time and funds for research or teaching endeavors. Clinicians at academic institutions, however, are still expected to produce scholarly work and must find time do so outside of their expected clinical duties.

In addition, the path to promotion based on recognition of clinical excellence alone is much harder to define than the other academic tracks. As a result, many clinicians remain at the assistant professor level, which is associated with less salary and sometimes less recognition from peers.

OTHER MATTERS

Health Care Management: Financial Pressures, Work Relative Value Units, and their Implications

---

Healthcare as a whole is an ever-changing industry manipulated by insurance practices and funding. In academic medicine faculty burnout stems from the gradual increase in workload as healthcare facilities struggle to maintain profit margins and remain competitive in a highly regulated industry. These stresses have direct impact on the day to day clinical operations including faculty productivity measures and administrative time. Productivity is measured by wRVUs which are driven by physician billing. So, the more patients in and out of the clinic the more wRVUs generated. Additionally, many hospitals are holding faculty accountable for quality measures and while these practices are generally valued by faculty and should be a standard part of the medical visit, these measures demonstrate that as more work is done in less time, quality must not suffer. Faculty now work longer hours and struggle to provide quality care with less face-to-face time with patients. And to keep things lean, incremental support staff is hard to come by despite the clinical growth.

For the medical center it can be a tough balance, as the same missions that draw clinicians to academic medicine, and away from greater compensation in community practice, are also more costly to the business. Neither research nor academics are as lucrative as clinical practice. For this reason, it can be a struggle to receive protected time to teach or conduct research. Academic institution should recognize these missions as long term investments. Research and education are what build the reputation for many of the academic medical centers across the country, a reputation that inevitably drives their clinical and financial growth.

—Comments from a rheumatology administrator at an academic institution.

Wickersham and colleagues[14] noted that although academic rheumatologists struggle to meet metrics that their clinical salaries are contingent on, they are a bargain for their institutions because they generate more than $10 for every $1 they receive for an office visit in the form of downstream revenue generated (eg, from imaging and laboratory tests). Every professional fee dollar charged by a rheumatologist for a visit with a patient with rheumatoid arthritis results in 20-fold to 30-fold additional charges for the institution. It would be a timely intervention to use some of the downstream revenue generated from rheumatology-based patient care toward supporting the academic missions of the faculty working in these institutions.

Professional Development

Recredentialing and maintenance of certification

Because academic rheumatologists are responsible for the care of complex patients and educating trainees, it is essential that they maintain their clinical knowledge and continue efforts for practice improvement. The results of a recent ACR survey revealed, however, that more than 90% of respondent rheumatologists believed that the current methods for maintenance of certification are too costly, cumbersome, and irrelevant. Another survey of US physicians showed that only 28% of physicians agreed that maintenance of certification activities were relevant to their patients and 81% believed they were a burden.[15]

To publish or perish

Publishing is important not only to share research findings but also to obtain national recognition and thus foster career advancement. Many academic institutions place great emphasis on the publication record during the promotion process, because dissemination of knowledge is one of the core missions of scholarly activity. As with extramural grant funding, however, publication in academic journals is highly competitive, with many top tier journals accepting less than 10% of submissions. To fill this void, there has been a huge expansion of lower-quality and even so-called predatory publishers that charge a significant fee for publication while bypassing traditional norms of peer review.

Professional societies—membership and volunteering

Professional societies are always in need of volunteers to help organize their annual meetings, workshops, continuing medical education courses, and legislative committees. This allows faculty an invaluable opportunity to take part in leadership positions, develop important organization skills, and connect with colleagues in the field.

Also, the opportunity to speak at national conferences or run workshops is important to build a regional and national reputation crucial for promotion.

There is stiff competition, however, when it comes to selection to these committees or for speaker invitations. Junior faculty who are not well recognized and do not already have committee or speaking experience tend to get passed over for more established faculty. The role of mentors and senior colleagues may be crucial to create opportunities for the next generation of rheumatologists to participate. Also, more formal vetting and evaluation of volunteer applications by selection committees are needed to make the selection process fairer.

Mentorship

As the demands of clinical medicine have changed and time is limited, volunteer mentoring has become more and more difficult for physicians. I will always mentor trainees because I truly get a great amount of satisfaction out of the process. I am fortunate to have had amazing mentors and I see it as my duty to "pay it forward."

—Comments from a clinical mentor at an academic center.

Effective mentorship is crucial for attracting the future generation of rheumatologists and for the survival and success of current ones. A mentor acts as a role model and an advocate for mentees, helping them set goals and providing them with networking and other opportunities that facilitate both professional and personal development.

Mentorship can take several forms, such as a traditional one-on-one relationship with a supervisor or as part of a larger program that incorporates professional development workshops, career planning, counseling, formal mentoring, and community network building. Studies of academic faculty have shown that effective mentorship leads to more productive faculty, earlier promotion, career satisfaction, and higher faculty retention.[16] In a study exploring the characteristics of successful and failed mentoring relationships conducted through the Departments of Medicine at the University of Toronto and University of California, it was found that successful relationships were characterized by reciprocity, mutual respect, clear expectations, personal connection, and shared values. Failed mentoring relationships were characterized by poor communication, lack of commitment, personality differences, perceived (or real) competition, conflicts of interest, and the mentor's lack of experience.[17] Mentees may struggle to find mentors in their particular area of interest from within their institution but reaching out to mentors from other institutions within or outside of the city may increase their chances of success.

One of the major barriers to building a successful mentor-mentee relationship or to attending professional development workshops is lack of time and financial support. Both parties have administrative, teaching, and clinical responsibilities and in addition a mentor often has to distribute their limited time between multiple other mentees. With the incorporation of the business model in medicine, there is now more emphasis on generating revenue from clinical activities, which means less time and financial resources for mentorship, teaching, and research.

Finally, the rheumatology community should strive to address the need to have an increasingly diverse group of mentors that reflect the diversity of mentees and to provide formal training programs that teach the skills required for effective mentorship.

Leadership

Strong leaders are essential for faculty career development and retention because they facilitate interinstitutional educational and research collaborations, champion faculty causes within the institution and at the national level.

Currently, there is a shortage of leaders in rheumatology and this is evident in (1) nonrheumatologists serving as division chiefs, (2) merger of entire rheumatology divisions into other subspecialties, and (3) the delay in hiring division chiefs despite aggressive advertising. Leaders in academic rheumatology also tend to be older, for example, the mean age of rheumatology division chiefs was 58 in 2012. Given the changing demographics of the rheumatology workforce, which are projected to comprise more minorities and women (57% of adult rheumatologists will be women in 2020),[1] leadership development needs to be purposefully inclusive of these groups. Multiple studies have shown that women faculty in medical schools do not feel accepted or supported to succeed and this is reflected by the absence or low numbers of women faculty in leadership positions.[9]

To ensure a robust supply of future division chiefs, fellowship directors, and college leaders, academic rheumatology centers need to actively engage and invest in the personal, professional, and leadership development of their academic faculty.

SUMMARY

The mission of academic institutions is threatened by increasing financial pressures and regulatory burdens. This has led to academic physicians spending more time generating wRVUs and less time pursuing the clinical excellence, quality education, and innovative research that are so valuable to patients and society.

It is increasingly important to acknowledge and address the challenges that have arisen for academic physicians, especially now, dealing with higher levels of physician burnout and the need to prevent further attrition of an already limited academic workforce.

Partnership between academic institutions, medical schools, professional organizations, and federal agencies is required to revitalize the academic mission and find innovative solutions to the problems faced by those in academics.

Such strategies might include formal mentorship and leadership training programs, new funding mechanisms to help researchers, redistribution of downstream revenues, less regulatory burden, and a more clearly defined academic pathway program for all those involved in academic medicine.

REFERENCES

1. Battafarano DF, Ditmyer M, Bolster MB, et al. 2015 American College of Rheumatology Workforce Study: supply and demand projections of adult rheumatology workforce, 2015-2030. Arthritis Care Res 2018;70(4):617–26.
2. Myasoedova E, Crowson CS, Kremers HM, et al. Is the incidence of rheumatoid arthritis rising?: results from Olmsted County, Minnesota, 1955-2007. Arthritis Rheum 2010;62(6):1576–82.
3. American College of Rheumatology. 2015 workforce study of rheumatology specialists in the United States. 2016. Available at: https://www.rheumatology.org/portals/0/files/ACR-Workforce-Study-2015.pdf. Accessed October 8, 2018.
4. Straus SE, Straus C, Tzanetos K, et al. Career choice in academic medicine: systematic review. J Gen Intern Med 2006;21(12):1222–9.
5. Grischkan J, George BP, Chaiyachati K, et al. Distribution of medical education debt by specialty, 2010-2016. JAMA Intern Med 2017;177(10):1532–5.
6. Ogdie A, Shah AA, Makris UE, et al. Barriers to and facilitators of a career as a physician-scientist among rheumatologists in the US. Arthritis Care Res (Hoboken) 2015;67(9):1191–201.
7. The state of women in academic medicine: the pipeline and pathways to leadership, 2015-2016. Available at: https://www.aamc.org/members/gwims/statistics/#tables. Accessed October 8, 2018.
8. Davidson A, Polsky D. Sustaining the rheumatology research enterprise. Arthritis Care Res 2015;67(9):1187–90.
9. NIH research portfolio online reporting tools - average age of principal investigators. Available at: https://search.usa.gov/search?utf8=%E2%9C%93&affiliate=ds_report&query=age+distribution+of+investigators&commit.x=0&commit.y=0. Accessed October 8, 2018.
10. NIH research portfolio online reporting tools - research project success rates by type and activity for 2017. Available at: https://report.nih.gov/success_rates/Success_ByActivity.cfm.
11. Nicholson LM, Schwirian PM, Groner JA. Recruitment and retention strategies in clinical studies with low-income and minority populations: progress from 2004-2014. Contemp Clin Trials 2015;45(Pt A):34–40.
12. Lawrence-Wolff K, Hildebrand B, Monrad S, et al. 2015 ACR/ARHP Workforce Study in the United States: A Maldistribution of Adult Rheumatologists [abstract]. Arthritis Rheumatol 2016;68(suppl 10). Available at: https://acrabstracts.org/abstract/2015-acrarhp-workforce-study-in-the-united-states-a-maldistribution-of-adult-rheumatologists/. Accessed October 9, 2018.

13. Sinsky C, Colligan L, Li L, et al. Allocation of physician time in ambulatory practice: a time and motion study in 4 specialties. Ann Intern Med 2016;165(11): 753–60.
14. Wickersharn P, Golz D, West SG. Clinical academic rheumatology: getting more than you pay for. Arthritis Rheum 2005;53(2):149–54.
15. Cook DA, Blachman MJ, West CP, et al. Physician attitudes about maintenance of certification. Mayo Clin Proc 2016;91(10):1336–45.
16. Sambunjak D, Straus SE, Marusic A. Mentoring in academic medicine: a systematic review. JAMA 2006;296(9):1103–15.
17. Straus SE, Johnson MO, Marquez C, et al. Characteristics of successful and failed mentoring relationships: a qualitative study across two academic health centers. Acad Med 2013;88(1):82–9.

Challenges of Practicing Rheumatology in a Government Setting

A County Hospital and Veterans Affairs Hospital Perspective

Gopika D. Miller, MD[a],*, Jasvinder A. Singh, MD, MPH[b]

KEYWORDS

- Rheumatology practice • Public sector rheumatology • VA rheumatology
- County rheumatology

KEY POINTS

- Per 2014 an American College of Rheumatology Benchmark Survey, only 2.6% of rheumatologists surveyed practice in a government setting.
- Veterans Affairs health systems as well as county health systems constitute government practice settings.
- Access to care, clinic structure, and access to biologic therapies are unique for rheumatology patients receiving care in a government setting.

INTRODUCTION

Recent data from the 2015 American College of Rheumatology and American Rheumatology Health Professionals workforce study project a rheumatology workforce shortage by 2030. According to available data, there are currently distinct changes noted within the rheumatology workforce (eg, number of full-time rheumatologists, shifting gender balance) and a real concern regarding the looming shortage of rheumatologists when the workforce data are projected to 2030.[1,2] Additional details

Grant Support: No funding support was obtained for this work. J.A. Singh is supported by the use of facilities at the Birmingham VA Medical Center, Birmingham, Alabama, USA.
Disclosure Statement: See last page of the article.
The views expressed in this article are those of the authors and do not necessarily reflect the position or policy of the Department of Veterans Affairs or the United States government.
[a] Division of Rheumatology, Los Angeles Biomedical Research Institute, Harbor-UCLA Medical Center, 1000 W. Carson Street, Box 470, Torrance, CA 90509, USA; [b] Musculoskeletal Outcomes Research, University of Alabama School of Medicine, 510, 20th Street South, Faculty Office Tower, Room 805 B, Birmingham, AL 35294-000, USA
* Corresponding author.
E-mail address: gopika.miller@gmail.com

Rheum Dis Clin N Am 45 (2019) 39–51
https://doi.org/10.1016/j.rdc.2018.09.004
0889-857X/19/© 2018 Elsevier Inc. All rights reserved.
rheumatic.theclinics.com

regarding the workforce shortage are highlighted in a separate Adam Kilian and colleagues' article, "Workforce Trends in Rheumatology," in this issue.

Based on data from the American College of Rheumatology Benchmark Tool, which collected survey information from 682 rheumatologists from 2012 to 2014, 3.1% of survey respondent rheumatologists reported employment in a government setting with 2.6% of those 3.1% who reported working in a government clinical setting (Veterans Affairs [VA]) as their primary practice setting[3] whereas the remaining 0.5% reported nonclinical work in a government setting (**Box 1, Fig. 1**). It is unclear if the participants were solicited via mail and/or electronic mail to participate in the survey because VA email addresses have been updated in recent years, so it is hard to know if adequate numbers of rheumatologists practicing in a government setting were reached for survey. Additionally, it is difficult to determine whether the survey accurately reflects the number of rheumatologists working in a government setting; for example, a public hospital system funded by state and federal funding or in a VA hospital and clinic setting. Many rheumatologists in these settings may have a dual appointment with the academic affiliate and, depending on the effort distribution for the clinical work, may select one versus the other site as the primary work setting.

We review the challenges and opportunities of working in a government setting by providing the perspective of the VA experience as well as the county/public hospital experience from Los Angeles County Department of Health Services (LAC DHS). LAC DHS is the second largest municipal health system in the United States and serves as an example of a large public hospital system.[4] We were asked to provide a perspective highlighting our experiences from our home county hospital and our home VA facility. We are fully aware that the experience from 1 county or 1 VA hospital cannot be generalized to other county or VA hospitals, respectively. VA and county medical centers vary in their size, structure, challenges, opportunities, and operations.

Box 1
Primary employment setting for survey respondents

Breakdown of the survey respondents practice setting

35.7%—Academic medical center

19.3%—Multispecialty group practice

16.4%—Single specialty group practice

15.3%—Solo practice

5.5%—Hospital-based practice

2.6%—Government clinical setting (Veterans Affairs)

1.5%—Other clinical setting

1.5%—Biomedical industry

1.4%—Retired

0.5%—Government nonclinical setting

0.5%—Other nonclinical setting

From Flood J. ACR's benchmark tool quantifies data about rheumatology workforce, clinical practice. The Rheumatologist. 2014. Available at: https://www.the-rheumatologist.org/article/acrs-benchmark-tool-quantifies-data-about-rheumatology-workforce-clinical-practice/. Accessed May 30, 2018.

Breakdown of practice activities and practice settings

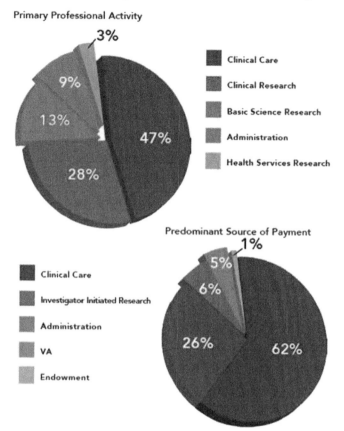

Primary Professional Activity

3%
9%
13%
47%
28%

- Clinical Care
- Clinical Research
- Basic Science Research
- Administration
- Health Services Research

Predominant Source of Payment

1%
5%
6%
26%
62%

- Clinical Care
- Investigator Initiated Research
- Administration
- VA
- Endowment

Fig. 1. American College of Rheumatology benchmarking tool. (*From* Flood J. ACR's benchmark tool quantifies data about rheumatology workforce, clinical practice. The Rheumatologist. 2014. Available at: https://www.the-rheumatologist.org/article/acrs-benchmark-tool-quantifies-data-about-rheumatology-workforce-clinical-practice/. Accessed May 30, 2018.)

We aim to highlight processes and services that are unique to practicing in a government setting to expand the reader's understanding of this practice setting and to underscore the need to serve this patient population on the state and national levels.

OVERVIEW OF RHEUMATOLOGY PRACTICE IN A GOVERNMENT SETTING

The practice of rheumatology in a government setting is unique. At LAC DHS, patients are seen for specialty care in the hospital-based rheumatology clinics that are located on the campuses of the 4 designated county hospitals. Based on their geographic data, patients are usually assigned to specific hospitals and hospital-based clinics for health services, but can be seen at any of the LAC DHS hospitals should they require services that are unavailable at their home institution. New patient referrals to rheumatology are generated from primary care clinics using an electronic referral system unique to LAC DHS (from both outlying county clinics as well as from hospital-based clinics), and from the emergency department and urgent care.

Uninsured patients make up about 10% of total ambulatory care visit volume in LAC DHS (Brad Spellberg, M.D, personal communication, 2018 with LAC USC Chief Medical Officer), which poses a unique challenge when considering access to care, diagnostics, and therapeutics. The mission of LAC DHS is "to ensure access to high-quality, patient-centered, cost-effective health care to LAC residents through direct services at DHS facilities and through collaboration with community and university partners."[4] Published data are not available that detail the total number of unique patient visits per year for ambulatory care nor is there further stratification of data for particular subspecialty services at each major clinical site or across the health system.

The VA is the largest, integrated, national health care system that provides care to US veterans.[5] At many VA medical centers, rheumatologists split their efforts between the VA and the academic affiliate and will perform clinical work, education, and/or research at both sites. Typically, patients referred to specialty care in the VA system are referred by their primary care doctors and then their referrals reviewed internally by the specialty reviewer (usually the clinical chief or the service chief for each specialty service) through the state-of-the-art electronic health record system, called the Computerized Patient Record System, which has been in use since 1998. The general themes for specialty care services provided at the VA, including rheumatology, are to provide high-quality, timely, efficient, and effective health care to veterans (**Box 2**).

Structure of the Los Angeles County Department of Health Services Rheumatology Clinics

Daily specialty clinics are not available for rheumatology services at LAC DHS. Patients have access to 3 allotted rheumatology clinic sessions. Clinics are specialized, such as, rheumatoid arthritis or lupus clinics, so patients essentially have access to their rheumatology clinic for 1 clinic session per week.

Owing to limitations with space, ancillary staffing constraints, and general resources, the LAC DHS clinics are not poised for increased capacity. New patient wait times are about 3 to 4 months for the initial rheumatology consultation unless the case seems to require urgent evaluation per the discretion of the electronic referral subspecialty reviewer for rheumatology, which can be expedited to a 2-week wait time.

Follow-up appointments for routine rheumatologic disease monitoring, in a patient with stable disease, are available typically every 4 months. Patients with higher

---

Box 2
Structure of clinics in a government setting

Access to care

- Daily rheumatology clinics are not available at LAC DHS.

- Daily rheumatology clinics are available at some VA medical centers.

- New patient referral wait time is 3 to 4 months at LAC DHS, and is usually <30 days at the VA.

- LA County rheumatology clinics depend on house staff with attending supervision for clinics to function.

- The VA rheumatology clinics are staffed by attendings or rheumatology fellows (or rarely mid-level practitioners) supervised by the attending physician.

Abbreviations: LAC DHS, Los Angeles County Department of Health Services; VA, Veterans Affairs.

disease activity or disease flares can be overbooked at a shorter time interval. Patients who are too sick to wait for their outpatient follow-up or procedure routinely present to the urgent care or the emergency department (data about total patient volume not available).

Because the LAC DHS hospitals and clinics provide patient care through collaboration with their community and university partners, the specialty clinics are staffed by house staff (postgraduate year [PGY]1 to PGY5), consisting of rotating rheumatology fellows and residents from family medicine and internal medicine. Variable staffing impacts the total volume of patients seen per day because house staff physicians are the main patient care providers in the subspecialty clinics at the LAC DHS rheumatology clinics. There is not adequate space nor ancillary staffing to allow for attending physician clinics to run in parallel with the house staff clinical activities. The attending physician reviews and supervises patient care with respect to review of pertinent data, provides teaching about rheumatologic diseases, assists with medical decision making, and supervises in-office procedures.

Structure of Veterans Affairs Rheumatology Clinics

New patient referral requests to the rheumatology service are generated through the electronic health record by primary care physicians or other specialists and are reviewed by the rheumatology service chief or clinical chief, usually within 2 business days. The rheumatology clinic templates are created based on the location of the VA, clinic setup, and full-time equivalent (FTE) rheumatologists. Typically, the rheumatology clinics are run by rheumatology attendings. In the university-affiliated VA medical centers, rheumatology clinics are staffed by the rheumatology fellows, PGY4 to PGY5 (and occasionally PGY1 to PGY3 house staff), or rarely medical students, who are supervised by rheumatology consultant/attendings.

At the VA clinics, there is a 30-day rule for a veteran to be scheduled for a clinic visit with any specialist care from the day of referral unless patient refuses or cancels or reschedules to a more convenient time. Recent institution of the Veterans Choice Program gives veterans the option to see a non-VA community provider/specialist closer to their residence who participate in the VA Veterans Choice Program network, if they (1) live far from the VA medical center providing their specialty services, (2) face excessive burden in traveling to the nearest VA medical facility, or (3) cannot get an appointment within 30 days of the clinically indicated date. Veterans must receive prior authorization from the VA to use the Veterans Choice Program, and expenses are paid by the VA.

There is variability of the number of clinic rooms and clinic staffing across various VA sites nationally. At most sites, the general use clinic space is shared and is used by the health care providers, nursing staff, and ancillary staff. The rheumatology clinic does not have designated nursing staff (or a nurse in charge). The shared space model can impact the total volume of patients seen per day given constraints on resource availability. In-clinic wait times at the VA clinics can vary across sites depending on the number of patients versus the number of providers/clinics, but the goal is usually less than 30 minutes.

Scope of services provided

- LAC DHS and VA clinics do not have capacity to care for patients with fibromyalgia nor osteoarthritis on a long-term basis.
- Primary care requests/general health maintenance occur frequently in county and VA clinic visits.

- Up to 10% of outpatient visits at LAC DHS are for uninsured patients after the institution of the Affordable Care Act.
- Inpatient rheumatology consult services are provided at LAC DHS and at the VA.

Los Angeles County Department of Health Services Rheumatology Clinic Services

Owing to the limited capacity of the LAC DHS rheumatology clinics, fibromyalgia and osteoarthritis management are deferred to primary care and/or orthopedics clinics for end-stage/late-stage osteoarthritis, or addressed primarily using the rheumatology e-consult platform to provide a treatment plan. The LAC DHS rheumatology clinics do not provide primary care services, such as diabetes management or routine health maintenance.

Many uninsured patients who do not have primary care providers use the county outpatient clinics (~10% visits). Since the institution of the Affordable Care Act, patients in the county system are assigned to or in the process of being assigned to primary care providers (data unavailable), yet their insurance plans tend to change sometimes on a monthly basis leading to gaps in access to care to primary care providers. This process leaves some patients who are seen for routine care in rheumatology specialty clinics with the possibility of being without a primary care provider, resulting in the rheumatology clinic appointment being used as a general health appointment, further increasing the complexity of the office visit.

The bulk of rheumatology services in the county setting are outpatient visits. Inpatient rheumatology consult services at each of the 3 county hospitals assist with the diagnosis and management of complex rheumatic conditions and complications.

Veterans Affairs Rheumatology Clinic Services

Most major VA centers have partial to 1 full rheumatology FTE, with very few centers with more than 1 FTE. For the roughly 140 VA Medical centers, there are approximately 113 FTEs for rheumatology, leading to an average of 1.03 rheumatologist per medical center (calculated by taking the total clinical workforce = 112.74/#sites with Rheum = 109) and 1.79 rheumatologist per 100,000 patients (personal communication, 2018 with Eileen Moran, Director VHA Office of Productivity Efficiency & Staffing New Haven, CT). This translates into 9.92 rheumatologists per 10,000 rheumatology patients. Long-term management of mechanical low back pain, fibromyalgia, and primary osteoarthritis are typically deferred to primary care owing to limited capacity. However, e-consults and 1-time rheumatology evaluations for diagnosis confirmation and/or advice regarding treatment plans are provided to the referring physician, who then assumes the long-term care of their mechanical low back pain, fibromyalgia, and osteoarthritis.

Even though rheumatology clinics are not designed to provide primary care services, veterans who receive ongoing care from the rheumatology service for disease management may see their rheumatologist 2 to 4 times per year versus seeing their primary care physician once a year (on average), despite a high comorbidity load. Owing to better access for veterans to rheumatology compared with primary care clinics, the rheumatologist often supplements primary care services in the spirit of service and patient convenience. The addition of nonrheumatologic care work is not usually captured for productivity units for work credit. However, it likely improves the quality of VA care being received by veterans who are seen at the VA specialty clinics, particularly in rheumatology. Inpatient services are available and consult requests are managed by the inpatient rheumatology consult services, similar to that described elsewhere in this article for the LA county hospitals.

Advantages and challenges of the government practice setting

- Advantages: Rapid access to biologics at low cost; VA electronic medical record/data collection; capacity to have registries and clinical study populations
- Challenges: Safety net patient population; high comorbidity burden; inadequate nursing and ancillary support

Veterans Affairs Perspective

Veterans have more chronic illnesses than the age- and sex-matched general US population.[6,7] Thus, the VA health care system serves as a safety net for a vulnerable population,[8,9] with a triple mission of patient care, education/training of health care providers through residency/fellowship training, and veteran-centered research on topics unique to or with heavy disease burden on veterans.

There are several advantages of practicing in the VA health care system that are evident. First, the well-established comprehensive electronic health record implemented in the VA system allows streamlined health care provision and enables rapid, efficient communication between rheumatologists (and other specialists) and other health care providers because everyone uses the same platform and can access records from other sites, either instantaneously or in a short time period with a request for records. Second, veterans have a very high show rate for their clinic follow-up visits, likely related to their trust in the VA health care system, recognition of provision of high-quality health care, and their respect for time, similar to their conduct during their military service. Third, the MyHealthEvet patient portal provides veterans with the ability to message their health care teams directly, obviating the need for a clinic visit or a long telephone call. Fourth, the VA has a streamlined drug formulary system that eliminates the lengthy preapproval process that is mandatory outside the VA system for approval of various treatments,[10] including biologic disease-modifying antirheumatic drugs (DMARDs).

The VA rheumatology service manages complex rheumatic diseases in veterans, including the use of immunosuppressive medications and biologics, as well as intravenous infusion of the biologics in the infusion centers, similar to the oncology service. High comorbidity burden in veterans with coexisting cardiac, renal, hepatic, pulmonary, and psychiatric diseases, makes the treatment with these agents more challenging and changes the risk/benefit ratio, compared with the healthy individuals who participate in clinical trials, and to the age-matched general US population, who have better health status, fewer comorbidities, and lower health care resource use.[7] A lack of adequate support from nursing and ancillary staff is a major limitation for the provision of rheumatologic care in the VA health care system, which was also recognized as a major contributor to delay in accessing care by veterans.

County Perspective

The advantage of practicing rheumatology in a county setting is that it allows the physician to be engaged in the care of rheumatologic diseases of a vulnerable patient population who are in the need of access to specialty care with a minimal caseload of soft tissue rheumatism/primary osteoarthritis and fibromyalgia. Additionally, the patients typically are presenting with severe disease manifestations and/or high disease activity, because the LAC DHS hospitals are urban safety net facilities. Another advantage is that the clinics are set up by disease state, which streamlines teaching/house staff education. By concentrating disease states in specific clinics, there is an improved opportunity for patient education and screening of the patients for potential recruitment to clinical studies. As part of their care team, the rheumatologists have a unique opportunity to make a dramatic impact in these patient's lives because they otherwise do not have access to routine or subspecialty care services based on either lack of insurance or underpowered/undervalued insurance. When patients who are routinely seen in the county rheumatology subspecialty clinics have attempted to transition to the private sector, the patients are typically referred back to the county system owing to low reimbursements for the private rheumatologist, high complexity of their case, and/or difficulty for the private rheumatologist to access advanced therapeutics and additional subspecialty expertise for their complex, ill, and underinsured patients.

There are unique challenges to practicing in a county setting. The main challenges center around access to the clinic space and ancillary staff for clinical care. Sporadic staffing and ancillary support in the clinical care areas leads to care delivery falling into the hands of the physicians and house staff, ranging from rooming the patients to transporting a patient to an urgent diagnostic study. Owing to the nature of using a shared clinic space, there is inconsistent staffing and clinic procedures and work flow inefficiencies. Although LAC DHS has a patient portal (started in 2015) to provide patients online access to their upcoming appointments and test results, less than 20% of the LAC DHS patients have routine access to a computer or the Internet. Of those patients who may have access to the Internet, they do not all speak English as a first language. In LAC DHS rheumatology clinics, up to 80% of patients are non-English speaking (with Spanish being the highest represented non-English language), which can pose a challenge to English-speaking physicians and care teams. Access to the infusion center is very limited, and the wait time is 4 weeks for a first available infusion chair, which can lead to admissions to the chemotherapy ward to provide patients with infusion treatments that they are unable to access in a timely fashion on an outpatient basis. In 2015, the LAC DHS hospitals successfully rolled out their electronic health record that connects inpatient and hospital-based outpatient care across the county. The disadvantage of the county's electronic health record is that it is does not communicate with local major hospitals such as UCLA, Kaiser, and Cedars-Sinai, which are all on EPIC and can share information through the CareEverywhere tab. The distinct county electronic health record could lead to fragmentation/separation of the care provided to an LAC DHS patient from the other major institutions/health systems within the county. The VA health system has its own unique electronic health record, which has functions that allow the users to view patient care records from other VA sites.

PATIENT-CENTERED CARE WITH ACCESS TO ADVANCED MEDICATIONS AND INFUSION THERAPIES

- Pharmacy-based protocol for medication order, approval, and delivery to the patient
- No prior authorization forms/paper work
- Timely access to conventional synthetic and biological DMARDs
- Infusion centers with limited resources/staffing can lead to hospitalization to expedite access to infusion therapy

Los Angeles County Department of Health Services

At the LAC DHS, the central pharmacy works in close collaboration with rheumatology prescribers to facilitate ease of access to therapeutics for rheumatology patients. There are no restrictions on conventional synthetic DMARD prescriptions when ordered by rheumatologists. As of 2018, there is no prior authorization form needed to prescribe adalimumab if you are a dermatologist, rheumatologist, or gastroenterologist. The adalimumab is simply ordered and the patient receives the medication from the county pharmacy at an extremely discounted rate; for example, adalimumab is 2 cents (personal communication with PharmD LAC DHS pharmacy; prices are subject to change based on annual negotiations with LAC DHS pharmacy).

In terms of access to non–tumor necrosis factor biologic DMARDs, the LAC DHS pharmacy requires an online form to be completed in addition to the medication order that has a brief description of tumor necrosis factor failure and rationale for the new medication. The prescription and authorization form is reviewed by the LAC DHS central pharmacy, the medication is then approved within 1 to 2 business days, and is available for pick up at the hospital-based county pharmacy. The LAC DHS pharmacy is inclined to provide non–tumor necrosis factor biologic medications to its patients if prescribed by an authorized specialty physician based on the understanding that the physician is referencing current and evidence-based prescribing practices. Additionally, novel therapeutics are made available to patients in step with their availability after approval by the US Food and Drug Administration, providing a safety net patient population with access to cutting edge therapy. The LAC DHS pharmacy truly aims to be physician and patient friendly in providing access to therapeutics for its patients without jumping through a variety of hoops that may not be medically necessary, indicated, or beneficial to the patient in question. LAC DHS pharmacy has a mail order drug program to facilitate access to medications, including biologic therapies.

At this time, there is not a clear written policy from the LAC DHS pharmacy regarding the LAC DHS formulary that is readily accessible to the public, whereas the VA provides access to its national formulary and prescribing practices that is easily accessible online.

Veterans Affairs

The VA has a clear protocol to provide medications for veterans receiving care at VA medical centers for their rheumatic diseases. In fact, there is a VA pharmacy and formulary Internet website that is extremely transparent and available to all to review. This website allows open access to all pharmacy protocols and general prescribing practices, and one can search the website easily by medication name.[10]

Most veterans have low copayments for medications, clinic visits, and laboratory and radiologic tests, most with a health condition arising from or diagnosed during their active duty receive between 0% to 100% service connection designated for that health condition. Copayments are decreased related to the percent service connection, and a 50% or higher service connection leads to free health care and a low copayment for each medication prescription ($7, but usually <$11) for their service-connected condition indefinitely.

VA patients have streamlined access to their medications and refills. Most medications, including traditional medications and novel medications, are usually available at the VA pharmacy at the same time or within weeks after their availability in the US market after their approval by the US Food and Drug Administration. The medications are typically available sooner than if prescribed through a private health maintenance organizations and/or through private insurance. The VA pharmacy categorizes medications as formulary that only require VA physician prescription for filling and refilling (eg, all conventional synthetic DMARD prescriptions, or traditional cytotoxic drugs for lupus/vasculitis) versus nonformulary drugs. Nonformulary drugs are the drugs for specialty disorders (eg, biologics) that require a prescription and an electronic nonformulary request by the ordering VA specialist. The VA specifies the criteria for nonformulary eligibility and approvals and specific specialties that are authorized to request high-cost and/or high-risk drugs (related to monitoring for toxicity/adverse events) for their diseases. These nonformulary electronic requests specify the diagnosis, the failure/contraindication of traditional medicines, and the reason for the failure, and the length of anticipated therapy and are sent electronically by the specialist to the VA pharmacists who promptly review the requests.

Medications for rheumatic disease treatment can also be recommended by veteran's civilian rheumatologist.[11] In such a scenario, co-management of the patient's disease by the VA provider (usually a VA rheumatologist or a VA primary care physician) and the civilian rheumatologist can be done. The VA rheumatologist (or primary care provider) can electronically write the VA prescription for the medication prescribed by a veteran's civilian rheumatologist, when in agreement, because the prescribing VA physician is legally responsible. When not in agreement, as in any comanagement model, providers discuss and usually mutually agree to a treatment option deemed most appropriate for the treatment of each veteran.

RESEARCH OPPORTUNITIES

- The electronic health record at the VA is a rich resource for clinical and health services outcomes research.
- The VA has its own funding mechanism for research aligned with issues specific to veterans.
- Plans for the LAC DHS electronic record to serve as resource for health services outcomes research.
- Challenges include balancing service and research time, and fluidity of protected time.

The VA health care system, with its national network, large size, and more than 20 years of administrative, clinical, and pharmacy data captured from the electronic health record, serves as a rich resource for clinical research as well as health services and outcomes research.[12]

Similar to the National Institutes of Health, the VA independently funds research on topics aligned with health care issues specific to veterans, including VA quality improvement initiatives. The VA research services include, clinical, and basic science Research—the VA Health Services Research and Development, Clinical Science Research and Development, and Basic and Laboratory Research and Development merit review grant mechanisms.[13] Grants are usually 3 years in duration, although up to 4-year projects are allowed as long as they are under the budget limit. Similar to the National Institutes of Health Career Development Program, the VA offers a Career Award for young, promising researchers to launch their research careers. The local VA leadership will allot 25% to 75% protected time for research for each funded merit review award, depending on the medical center leadership and the number of grants. In addition to these awards, the VA also supports VA centers of excellence by providing support for a research core with related 2 to 3 research projects, called CREATE[14] and COIN,[15] both of which can be competitively renewed. The VA also supports Service Directed Projects, which are focused on testing clinical care initiatives, rather than having a pure research focus.[16] Several VA medical centers have a VA Quality Improvement (QI) Scholar Programs, that pair a young researcher interested in QI with mentor/

s and protects time over 1 to 3 years for completing a QI project. These research grants and QI mechanisms are a generous way to develop and nurture VA research careers and discover solutions for veteran health by providers who also provide care to veterans on a regular basis.

Challenges with balancing clinical services and renewing federal research grants

1. Issues with a fixed money pool and expanding number of researchers competing for the same pot of money;
2. Rapid change in areas of emphasis and priorities, in line with the political climates and new challenges;
3. An emphasis on having an implementation aspect to every research project, whether appropriate or not, because there is increasing unease in performing pure clinical or epidemiologic or health services research;
4. "Forgotten diseases" such as gout and osteoarthritis are funded at much lower proportional funds compared with cardiac, oncology, psychiatric, or procedure-related fields; and
5. The change in performance pay from a combination of research and clinical objectives previously to predominantly clinical goals is a challenge for a physician scientist salary parity.

County Setting

Health services research, and clinical and basic sciences research activities occur in the county setting. The majority of research performed is health services research and is supported when it aligns with county priorities. Based on individual physician investigator's interests, the investigator can have anywhere from 10% to 50% protected time for county-aligned research that must be approved by the department chair. The investigator could use an additional 24 hours of their personal time to reach 70% protected research time, as long as their research aligns with county priorities.

Allotted research time depends on the medical center, your hiring item/employment item, and university affiliation if any. Challenges often arise with balancing clinical services and service obligations, and securing grant funding. LAC DHS employees are employees of the county and thus have a service obligation to the county. If they would like to be physician scientists with an affiliation to the university or with a research institute, the rheumatologist either has to supplement their income from a private practice/relative value unit–based model or provide their entire income through grant funding, but they have hospital privileges to participate in clinical teaching/supervision.

SUMMARY

Practicing rheumatology in a government setting is challenging yet highly rewarding owing to unique opportunities that allow for high clinical impact in patient care, meaningful research data sources, and funding mechanisms and provision of timely and appropriate access to basic and advanced therapeutics, which are the cornerstone to chronic disease management in rheumatology.

DISCLOSURE STATEMENT

G.D. Miller: No disclosures. J.A. Singh has received consultant fees from Crealta/Horizon, Fidia, UBM LLC, Medscape, WebMD, the National Institutes of Health, and the American College of Rheumatology. J.A. Singh is a member of the Veterans

Affairs Rheumatology Field Advisory Committee. J.A. Singh is the editor and the Director of the UAB Cochrane Musculoskeletal Group Satellite Center on Network Meta-analysis. J.A. Singh served as a member of the American College of Rheumatology's (ACR) Annual Meeting Planning Committee (AMPC) and Quality of Care Committees, the Chair of the ACR Meet-the-Professor, Workshop and Study Group Subcommittee, and the co-chair of the ACR Criteria and Response Criteria subcommittee. J.A. Singh is a member of the executive of OMERACT, an organization that develops outcome measures in rheumatology and receives arms-length funding from 36 companies.

REFERENCES

1. Bolster MB, Bass AR, Hausmann JS, et al. 2015 American College of Rheumatology Workforce Study: the role of graduate medical education in adult rheumatology. Arthritis Rheumatol 2018;70(6):817–25.

2. Battafarano DF, Ditmyer M, Bolster MB, et al. 2015 American College of Rheumatology Workforce Study: supply and demand projections of adult rheumatology workforce, 2015-2030. Arthritis Care Res (Hoboken) 2018;70(4):617–26.

3. Flood J. ACR's benchmark tool quantifies data about rheumatology workforce, clinical practice. The Rheumatologist; 2014. Available at: http://www.the-rheumatologist.org/article/acrs-benchmark-tool-quantifies-data-about-rheumatology-workforce-clinical-practice. Accessed May 30, 2018.

4. Health Services Los Angeles County. About DHS. Available at: http://dhs.lacounty.gov/wps/portal/dhs/moredhs/aboutus. Accessed August 1, 2018.

5. Iglehart JK. Reform of the Veterans Affairs health care system. N Engl J Med 1996;335(18):1407–11.

6. Singh JA, Borowsky SJ, Nugent S, et al. Health-related quality of life, functional impairment, and healthcare utilization by veterans: veterans' quality of life study. J Am Geriatr Soc 2005;53(1):108–13.

7. Agha Z, Lofgren RP, VanRuiswyk JV, et al. Are patients at Veterans Affairs medical centers sicker? A comparative analysis of health status and medical resource use. Arch Intern Med 2000;160(21):3252–7.

8. Wilson NJ, Kizer KW. The VA health care system: an unrecognized national safety net. Health Aff (Millwood) 1997;16(4):200–4.

9. Wolinsky FD, Coe RM, Mosely RR 2nd, et al. Veterans' and nonveterans' use of health services. A comparative analysis. Med Care 1985;23(12):1358–71.

10. VA National Formulary. Available at: https://www.data.va.gov/dataset/va-national-formulary. Accessed August 1, 2018.

11. Schwab P, Sayles H, Bergman D, et al. Utilization of care outside the veterans affairs health care system by US Veterans With Rheumatoid Arthritis. Arthritis Care Res (Hoboken) 2017;69(6):776–82.

12. Boyko EJ, Koepsell TD, Gaziano JM, et al. US Department of Veterans Affairs medical care system as a resource to epidemiologists. Am J Epidemiol 2000;151(3):307–14.

13. US Department of Veterans Affairs. Office of Research & Development. Available at: https://www.research.va.gov/. Accessed August 1, 2018.

14. US Department of Veterans Affairs. HSR&D Collaborative Research to Enhance and Advance Transformation and Excellence (CREATE) Initiative. Available at: https://www.hsrd.research.va.gov/centers/create/. Accessed August 1, 2018.

15. Health Services Research and Development. VA HSR&D centers. Available at: https://www.hsrd.research.va.gov/centers/default.cfm. Accessed August 1, 2018.
16. Health Service Research & Development. Service directed research (SDR). Available at: https://www.hsrd.research.va.gov/funding/sdr.cfm. Accessed August 1, 2018.

The Focused Musculoskeletal Factory

Gerald M. Eisenberg, MD

KEYWORDS

- Group practice • Private practice • Multispecialty practice

KEY POINTS

- Private practice models need to adapt to changing economic pressures.
- A one-stop comprehensive care setting for people with musculoskeletal disease is an attractive alternative for patients and payers alike.
- A physician-owned and directed multispecialty practice offers the rheumatologist professional satisfaction and enhanced financial opportunity.

BACKGROUND

The development and formalization of the practice of rheumatology has been a relatively recent development in comparison with most other areas of medical specialization. Board Certification in Rheumatology was not offered until 1972 and Fellowship in the American College of Rheumatology did not exist until 1986. Up until the turn of the 21st century, rheumatology was practiced overwhelmingly by small groups of 1 to 3 physicians in academic or community-based settings. Occasionally, some academic centers might have larger numbers of rheumatologists seeing patients, teaching, doing bench research, and participating in clinical trials. Larger numbers of rheumatologists practicing together was certainly the exception to the rule. Multiple factors have combined over the past 20 years, which have had a profound impact on how medicine, in general, as well as rheumatology, specifically, has been practiced. The revolution in our understanding of the immune response and our ability to impact on immune function gone wrong has literally revitalized the specialty of rheumatology since 2000. At exactly the same time, the "businessfication" of medicine has made the practice of a cognitive medical specialty increasingly more challenging, especially for the traditional model of the small rheumatology practice.[1] This issue of Rheumatic Disease Clinics is focused on various aspects of rheumatology practice and this particular review focuses on one approach to successfully dealing with the complex environment of 21st century rheumatology practice.

Disclosure Statement: The author has nothing to disclose.
Illinois Bone and Joint Institute, 9000 Waukegan Road, Morton Grove, IL 60053, USA
E-mail address: geisenberg@ibji.com

Rheum Dis Clin N Am 45 (2019) 53–66
https://doi.org/10.1016/j.rdc.2018.09.005
0889-857X/19/© 2018 Elsevier Inc. All rights reserved.

Successful medical practice remains, hopefully, centered around the relationship between the patient and his or her physician. However, there are other critical relationships that have come into play, which also must be navigated for a practice to prosper. Insurance companies and other payers, benefit management companies, hospital systems, state and federal government agencies, and employee relations all need to be competently addressed for a practice to grow and for its patients to be successfully treated. All of these additional players in medical care see their services as deserving of reimbursement and profitability and have no problem in generating those profits at the expense of the patient as well as the treating physician. To a certain extent, the growth of "medical business" has occurred in the relative vacuum of business expertise on the part of the traditional practicing physician. In the past 20 years, the explosive growth of the insurance industry, the consolidation of hospital systems nationwide, and the availability of extremely effective and extremely expensive treatments with the resulting bonanza of unheard of profitability for big pharmaceutical companies have all placed increasing financial pressure on doctors' practices. In addition, the business acumen accumulated over the past 25 years has enabled hospital systems, insurance companies, pharmacy companies, and private investors to become involved in the practice of medicine, sometimes leaving practicing physicians in the dust of limited time, resources, and strategic vision.[2]

As these major shifts in the finances and management of medical practice have occurred, the public's relationship with its medical care and doctors has also undergone seismic, and not necessarily positive, change. Increasing competition, decreasing physician reimbursement, expansion of marketing, and ever-increasing consumer expectations have placed medical practice under the same microscope as any other retail business. People want what they want when they want it and those practices that cannot deliver are finding that the traditional doctor–patient relationship does not always carry the day.

In the past 10 years physicians have been caught in the potential death spiral of decreasing reimbursement and increasing expenses. Employee salaries and benefits, the rent, the costs of equipment and furnishings, as well as professional liability insurance have not stood still. The government mandate for the electronic medical record, Health Insurance Portability and Accountability Act (HIPAA), insurance preauthorization for medications and procedures, and marketing are just a few examples of significant practice expenses that literally did not exist as recently as 10 years ago. So, doctors are being squeezed. This financial pressure is a root cause of the deterioration of the sacred relationship between the doctor and patient.[3] Doctors are no longer at the center of what has become a very complicated system of medical care. Others have seized this opportunity and we have paid for it.

NEW STRATEGIES FOR NEW CHALLENGES

In 1997, Regina Herzlinger, Professor of Business Administration at the Harvard Business School, authored Market Driven Healthcare, which was her attempt at addressing the increasingly competitive and increasingly consumer-driven world of health care and medical practice.[4] She expanded on the idea of finding the right "niche" in services and focusing on delivering the best possible care which would, of necessity, ultimately be the most cost-effective care as well. She referred to the "focused factory," a term that had been introduced in the mid-1970s and referred to manufacturing processes that focused on only one or a very few products and did it as well and efficiently as possible. She suggested that the focused medical factory could concentrate on one area of increasingly specialized medical care and do it better than others. In this way, such a practice could not only survive but flourish. There were already several well-known examples of these focused medical factories. The Mayo Clinic was established in the late 1880s when a small group of doctors combined their resources to provide comprehensive medical and surgical care, in one setting, to their patients. In the subsequent 135 years, the Mayo Clinic remains the prototypical large group practice, whose size and scope provide the resources for good patient care, physician education, and ongoing research.[5] The Hospital for Special Surgery in New York has a long and proud history of providing focused care specifically in the area of orthopedic care, research, and teaching. Since the Second World War, The Hospital for Special Surgery has also developed a successful and sophisticated rheumatology program, which, together with other musculoskeletal specialists, provides multidimensional care to people with musculoskeletal and autoimmune disease. But rheumatologists and orthopedists are acutely aware that close collaboration between the specialties is the exception, rather than the rule.

In the 1970s, Dr Daniel McCarty was the Director of Rheumatology at the University of Chicago and one of his faculty was Dr John Skosey. Dr Skosey has recalled that Dr McCarty frequently would comment on the positive impact on patient care that might ensue with close collaboration between orthopedists and rheumatologists. Dr McCarty suggested that close proximity of rheumatologists and orthopedists in the clinics would expedite and improve care (Dr John Skosey, personal communication, 2017). Dr Skosey kept this in mind when he arrived at the University of Illinois as Chief of Rheumatology in 1978. Within a few years he established multidisciplinary clinics with both dermatology and orthopedic surgery. In these combined clinics, patients with overlapping clinical issues would be seen simultaneously by the needed specialists. It was my good fortune to attend these multidisciplinary sessions as a rheumatology fellow and junior attending between 1979 and 1982. An additional participant in some of those years was an orthopedic resident, Dr Wayne Goldstein, who subsequently took additional training in joint replacement at the Brigham Hospital with Dr Clement Sledge.

PREDECESSORS TO THE "FOCUSED FACTORY"

Thereafter, I practiced rheumatology in a hospital-based multispecialty practice in the Chicago area. Our rheumatologists had active practices, interacted on a daily basis with medical students and residents and conducted clinical research, as a matter of routine. At the same time, Dr Goldstein returned to the Chicago area after his joint replacement fellowship in Boston and joined an orthopedic practice that was, coincidently, at the same hospital where I was a hospital-employed physician. Dr Goldstein and I renewed our old collegial relationship and actively referred patients to one another. We were, however, in separate locations and in separate practices. By the early 1990s, Dr Goldstein had refined his vision for comprehensive orthopedic care and recruited the first of several orthopedic subspecialists in hand as well as sports medicine. Over the next several years, spine, trauma, foot, and ankle were added to the practice roster. Dr Goldstein and his orthopedic partners were establishing a large and successful subspecialty orthopedic practice.

In the meantime, the hospital-based rheumatology practice I was part of grew from 2 to 6 rheumatologists and we expanded our scope of services to include not only traditional rheumatic disease, but osteoporosis as well. We were "given" a DXA machine in 1990 that had been underutilized in the hospital setting. In addition, 2 of us learned how to do epidural steroid injections for our older patients with lumbar stenosis. We were active teachers at the hospital and in the community and developed a reputation for delivering state of the art care. We ultimately convinced the hospital to allow us to establish a practice site, which was well removed from the hospital campus, where access was easy and rheumatology patients would not face the various inconveniences that came with visits on the hospital campus. This outpatient facility would have X ray, bone densitometry, laboratory services, and physical therapy, all in one setting. Office hours were expanded and we were the only rheumatologists in the area offering evening and Saturday office hours.

A lot of this changed when the hospital that employed us made some poor business decisions and found itself in financial stress in the mid-1990s. The hospital ultimately sought a partner in the Chicago area with which to merge and with that came a new and less physician-friendly atmosphere. There is no question that competition was ramping up amongst nascent hospital systems at that point and doctors were being referred to as "cost centers" and "profit centers" in meetings I personally attended. On top of that, it rapidly became clear that hospitals at that point were not good at managing doctors' practices. The close attention to nickels and dimes that had always been the hallmark of successful practice management was initially lost on the hospital systems that saw doctors and their practices as a marketing device and gateway to inpatient hospital care. The doctors, themselves, were at arm's length from the practice's financial performance, which they viewed as a "black box." One of the last straws for us was when hospital management closed the small outpatient physical therapy department we had developed at our office. We were told it was a "money loser." For me and my rheumatology partners, it was time to find a better way. (In an ironic twist, when the rheumatologists did leave the hospital's employ, the hospital sold the building where we had practiced, several miles away from the hospital campus. The building was torn down and replaced with a huge privately owned physical therapy facility!)

REALIZING THE MODEL

Although the hospital-based multispecialty practice had provided some outstanding advantages, compared with the smaller private practices in our area, none of us was interested in simply moving to another hospital system as employees. Our collegial relationship with Dr Goldstein and his partners had matured over the years. Dr Goldstein and I both recalled the combined ortho/rheum clinics we had attended almost 20 years earlier at the University of Illinois. Dr Goldstein proposed, and we accepted his suggestion, that our rheumatology practice fully merge into the orthopedic practice that was already known as The Illinois Bone and Joint Institute (IBJI).

I pause for a moment and ask the reader to do the same. For what I have just described was an extraordinary occasion. Dr Goldstein, who already had demonstrated the vision required to develop an orthopedic subspecialty practice (common now, not common then) had enthusiastically endorsed the idea of rheumatologists and orthopedists practicing together and using their combined skills to efficiently and successfully treat people with musculoskeletal disease. I submit that having an orthopedic champion for this model of care was the single most important factor in establishing this kind of practice. If not for his drive, I am doubtful that the merger would have been undertaken. There are now more than 100 physician members of IBJI and most of them take the presence of rheumatologists as a given, if not a true asset to their practice. Twenty years ago, however, there was plenty of doubt.

I was the first rheumatologist who joined IBJI in January of 1999 and was joined by 5 of my former group partners over the next 18 months. In another twist, we were ultimately joined in our practice by Dr John Skosey who, not surprisingly, found our model of practice extremely attractive! Working with my former chief has been a highlight in my career.

Conceptually, having rheumatologists and orthopedists working closely together with patients in common makes a lot of sense. As usual, the devil was in the details. How could we merge a high income, procedural specialty such as orthopedics with a lower income, cognitive medical specialty such as rheumatology? This model was almost unheard of in community-based, private practice. Although many university centers employed both orthopedists and rheumatologists, they rarely worked together, in the same space, on the same patients. University centers, especially in years past, maintained rigid silos where rheumatologists and orthopedists occupied very separate turf.

Although our long-standing collegial relationship initially launched the merged enterprise, it would ultimately be driven by the advantages offered by the group practice model. Group practice allows its physicians to develop ancillary services and to maximize negotiating leverage. If a group is big enough, services that are traditionally associated with the hospital can be offered to patients and those services can be offered at a price and level of convenience that simply cannot be met by a hospital system.[6] Ask any insurance company and they will agree. If a group is large enough and offers expertise in an area, such as musculoskeletal care, it is difficult, if not impossible, for payers to circumvent reasonable contracting terms with such an entity.

In respect to ancillary services, the rheumatologists already had experience with X ray, bone densitometry, laboratory services, and physical therapy. We had just begun infusion services for a year or so before our merger and had a vigorous clinical trials program. All of these services were brought to our new situation at IBJI. The orthopedists, of course, had x-ray services already. But these other ancillary services were new to them. Subsequently, IBJI has added MRI, occupational therapy, durable medical equipment, diagnostic and procedural ultrasound, and C-arm fluoroscopy for injections. It was our good fortune, and our patients' good fortune, that infusion therapy exploded at exactly the time that our practice merger took place. It remains an important patient service as well as an important ancillary activity.

There are certainly vibrant single specialty rheumatology practices that have developed some or all of the ancillary services mentioned. If the number of rheumatologists is large (compared with most rheumatology practices) this can be done. Having multiple orthopedic partners does, however, change the financial picture and allows the scale of the ancillaries to increase substantially. At this time, IBJI ancillary volume is considerable.

A NEW CULTURE

Having looked at other practice options at that time, we found the potential for multidisciplinary musculoskeletal care to be irresistible. The first question to be answered was whether the 2 "cultures," rheumatology and orthopedics, would be compatible in the private practice setting. The rheumatologists were initially most concerned that we would be looked down on by our orthopedic colleagues as someone less valuable than they. Income disparities between the 2 specialties were universally acknowledged, and the traditional hospital "pecking order" placed orthopedists at the center of the hospital universe with rheumatologists somewhere beyond Pluto. In our particular regard, the rheumatologists' clinical maturity and the simultaneous evolution of the medical environment from the hospital to the outpatient setting was helpful in leveling the playing field somewhat. All 6 of the rheumatologists who initially joined IBJI were very experienced clinicians with recognized expertise and large, established practices. A couple of us had served significant administrative and academic roles in our previous practice setting. By that point, we clearly understood the difference between being hospital/system employees and private practitioners and we were confident we could bring added value to the practice that would help differentiate IBJI from other orthopedic practices, both in the private and academic settings.

The question, of course, was whether our new orthopedic partners would see it the same way. In this way, we were clearly benefitted by the presence of Dr Goldstein, who was the president and founder of IBJI, as well as a seasoned clinician. He was, and remains, a respected voice amongst his orthopedic partners and pushed his partners, at that time, to see the bigger picture. Rightfully, several of the orthopedists at IBJI at that time were concerned that bringing in rheumatologists would be a drag on overhead. Rheumatologists spent all their time in the office, they did not operate, and they did not earn as much. How could they support the overhead of a large, orthopedic practice? How would having rheumatologists in the practice effect referral patterns? In addition, there were questions about personality fit. Fortunately, we were known entities to one another. On the balance, that was a positive situation, but there was still some hesitancy, from both sides, as to whether the 2 sides in the equation would match up.

Some of the nuts and bolts of the relationship would need to be answered immediately. The rheumatologists insisted, from the start, that the merger would result in full partnership after a reasonable period of time had passed. This turned out to be 2 years. Although it was true that our income potential was lower than our orthopedic partners, there were forces at play that were blunting the disparity. Procedural reimbursement was decreasing. Orthopedic practice was moving from the hospital to the outpatient surgery center and to the office. Income from office visits was an increasingly important factor for many orthopedists. We felt that rheumatologists in the practice could offset some of the fixed orthopedic overhead. When our ortho partners were in the operating room, the rheumatologists would be using empty office space to see patients. Infusion therapy, unknown to orthopedists, supplied a constant stream of patients to the practice. Not only was infusion therapy remunerative, but many of these same patients would choose to use IBJI orthopedists when surgical questions arose. Indeed, the whole notion of rheumatologists and orthopedists working together was predicated on timely and appropriate referrals between the 2 specialties that would optimize care and outcomes.

In addition to the increase in interaction between the 2 specialty groups, the other strong argument in favor of the pairing of the 2 groups was that it would make IBJI more distinctive than it had been previously. There was no practice in our area where a patient with any musculoskeletal question could get it answered in one place. We proposed that we were truly a "one-stop shop." We wanted our new orthopedic partners to embrace this; we wanted our other referring physicians to know this; we wanted chiropractors and other alternative health practitioners to know this; we wanted the payers to know this. But, most of all, we wanted the public to know this. The idea was that if you have a bone and joint question or problem, you just needed IBJI. It was the beginning of the era of decreased access to one's primary care physician and this message could have universal appeal.

COMPENSATION FORMULA

After initial negotiations, the compensation arrangements were clarified and agreed on. Compensation would be based on professional productivity. One's office collections would be the main driver of income, which would vary with volume. Ancillary income fell into 2 buckets. Rheumatology ancillaries were defined as those services used exclusively, or almost exclusively, by the rheumatologists. These included infusion, DXA, laboratory, and rheumatology clinical research. Each of these services would pay its overhead out of collections, with the remaining profits (or losses) split amongst the rheumatologists. The other ancillary bucket derived from those services used by rheumatologists and orthopedists, alike, and ultimately came to include physical/occupational therapy and MRI. Over the past 20 years, additional services have been added and the attribution of ancillary income has been modified from time to time,[7] but the basic formula has remained unchanged.

Determining group overhead (indirect expenses) is complex in any practice organization and IBJI is no exception. Rent, front desk, billing, "back office," answering service, and scores of other everyday expenses are allocated evenly across all members. Clinical staffing, liability insurance, and educational expenses were variable for each group member and were considered direct expenses. Overall rheumatology overhead was calculated at a fixed percentage above the indirect orthopedic overhead, because all rheumatology expenses and collections were generated in the office, whereas a significant percentage of orthopedic collections were generated in the operating room, with relatively less practice overhead. It seemed fair, from everyone's point of view, that completely office-based physicians should have an overhead percentage higher than physicians who generated some income elsewhere. The fact that rheumatology and orthopedic overhead were directly linked gave both groups "skin in the game" to keep expenses controlled.

Thus, a rheumatology compensation formula was derived, which was identical for all the rheumatologists, tied to our ortho partners' overhead, and driven, in the main, by our individual productivity. It has remained an agreement that most of us find acceptable.[8]

In discussing the compensation formula, the office-based nature of rheumatology has been emphasized. This has remained true over the last 20 years. Although we do see inpatients in consultation as well as our own patients when they are hospitalized, the yearly income derived from inpatient care is approximately 1% of total income for the rheumatologists.

GOVERNANCE AND ADMINISTRATION

With a compensation plan in place, next steps involved fully integrating our rheumatology practice into the governance of the merged musculoskeletal practice. To be frank, we understood that we were a half dozen rheumatologists merging with a much larger group of orthopedists. However, the 6 of us had significant involvement in group and hospital politics and group practice governance. We felt strongly we had something to contribute to the culture of an evolving musculoskeletal practice.[9] Early on, we had intuitively identified a small number of our new ortho partners who saw themselves as individual practitioners who did not depend on or require the support of any of their partners, orthopedic, rheumatologic, or otherwise. The evolution of IBJI's culture remains a work in progress to which the rheumatologists, despite our relatively small numbers, have contributed with gusto. Beyond clinical collaboration, the rheumatologists sit on the practice management committee, as well as other governance committees, such as marketing, ethics, operations, and others. Over time, our orthopedic partners have not only accepted our presence but also have ultimately welcomed it.

The rate of change in the practice of medicine continues to accelerate. Declining reimbursement; competition from systems; competition at the local pharmacy (I recall seeing a flyer from a local pharmacy "doc in the box" advertising screening for Lyme disease); the need to be HIPAA compliant; electronic medical records; prescription and procedural preauthorizations; and marketing in the press, radio, television, and social media have changed, in a fundamental way, how doctors practice. These modern realities play more easily into the group practice model. It is difficult, if not impossible, for many smaller medical practices to maintain themselves in this increasingly expensive atmosphere. Some practices have the wherewithal to charge its patients a premium, or membership, to support these onerous expenses. In some situations, physicians have opted out of the insurance rat race altogether and are run as cash businesses (such as your grocery store or your plumber).[10] More power to the physicians who can do it. But, as one of my partners said to me, about 10 years ago, "Who will take care of our parents? Who will be around to take care of US?"

Large group practices will likely be around.[11] They are more nimble than large systems that are accountable to a lay board or investors. The administrative structure that reports to a board or investors is, itself, an interest group that may consider physicians and even patients, secondarily. By definition, physician group practices are owned and directed by their physician members. That does not mean that they are necessarily figuring the budget or adjusting the heat, but they sign the checks and had better have significant input into strategic planning, major spending, the patient experience, the employee experience, and the wellbeing and retention of the physicians themselves. Who better than the doctors in the office seeing their patients to make these decisions?

These days, successful practices require all manner of administrative expertise to advance ambitious practice agendas. This starts with strong office management. The office administrator should ideally view her/himself as working for 2 bosses; the patient and the doctor. An effective administrator is able to communicate clearly, yet with empathy, with both parties, multiple times a day, while still dealing with staff who is late, supplies that do not arrive, medical emergencies that disrupt the best laid plans, and other daily drama. An effective administrator is an essential complement to physician governance, but does not replace it. Beyond the front desk, telecom, and clinical office support, a large group must support an increasingly sophisticated back office. At IBJI this includes a COO (nonphysician) who coordinates and implements group strategy as well as a CFO responsible for budget, prompt payment of group bills, and helping doctors to allocate limited financial resources. A good CFO is absolutely invaluable in clarifying for the physician members, in financial terms they can understand, just what is going on in their practice. In a group with many employees, human resources is occupied to a great extent by the usual comings and goings of employees, in-house health maintenance programs, employee satisfaction and grievances, and all manner of insurance questions. Risk management deals with group legal issues, medical liability, HIPAA, compliance, and contracting with payers. For the past 10 years our group has had fulltime information technology support in the office as well as remotely available to deal with our large electronic medical record, imaging picture archiving and communication system (PACS), and telephone issues. The practice supports a large billing function, which deals not only with billing and collections but accurate coding and documentation, as well.

Having real contracting expertise is a critical piece in making sure that the payers recognize the value of a skilled and large musculoskeletal practice. Payer contracting for a group with orthopedists, rheumatologists, podiatrists, physiatrists, as well as physical and occupational therapists is complicated. None of these groups will get top dollar for their services from the payers in every instance. It is the job of the person negotiating the contract to make sure that the group, overall, gets the best deal possible; this means close and cogent conversation with physician members to explain the overall impact of a contract. I would certainly not accuse insurance companies of being particularly obsessed with patient convenience, but having multiple services available in one outpatient setting for people with musculoskeletal disease is an attractive and increasingly cost-effective approach for payers and patients alike.

SIZE DOES MATTER

Hospitals have merged and formed systems that have purchased medical practices. Pharmaceutical companies have merged and merged again. Pharmacy companies have purchased insurance companies (and vice versa). Insurance companies have contracted with benefit management companies, then devoured those same benefit management companies. This has all been done to accomplish that elusive economy of scale and increase profitability. It is probably not coincidental that these same steps have reduced competition amongst these various entities.

So, it turns out that size does matter. A small practice can be ignored or marginalized by payers. It is unfortunately not rare for hospital systems to approach small specialty practices (cardiology is one good example) and make it "an offer they cannot refuse" to become hospital employed. The (usually) unspoken alternative is that the system will hire someone else, steer referrals to the new specialists, and put strong financial stress on the preexisting practice. The emerging practice expenses already sited, by themselves, can be enough to sink a small practice. In the Chicago area, several small rheumatology practices found that the expense of converting to an electronic medical record was an extreme financial pressure.

The migration of medical care from the hospital setting to the outpatient setting has the attention of the payers and the hospital systems. It is one of the major reasons that large, musculoskeletal group practice is increasingly more attractive. If there is enough volume, rheumatology patients can receive almost all of the care they require in the office, without the huge overhead of a hospital structure. Even joint replacement surgery is rapidly moving to the outpatient setting at a pace no one would have foreseen only 2 or 3 years ago. IBJI now has more than 15 office sites and offers rheumatologic care at 7 of them.

Economy of scale is not automatic, however. If costs and reimbursement are not carefully tracked, it does not take long to see margin disappear. This means that physician partners must be acutely aware of their own charges and collections and that relatively esoteric collection issues are not lost in the shuffle. In addition, there must be "group think" that allows for more global awareness of the ebb and flow of the larger practice. An example of this is infusion therapy. The cost of infusion drugs is one of IBJI's largest expenses. Yet, there is no margin to speak of on the medications, themselves. We essentially provide a "pass through" of the medication to the patient, at no profit, given our costs and reimbursement for infusion drugs. Initially, our orthopedic partners were nonplussed that IBJI was spending 7 figures yearly on drugs with no profit margin. Careful explanation from their rheumatology partners, however, showed how the infusion business worked and that there were substantial charges and collections for the professional services associated with the delivery of the drug, even if the expenses and profit on the drug itself was a wash.[12] There is now universal understanding in our group that infusion therapy is good for patients and good for IBJI, as well.

From time to time, issues arise about the cost-effectiveness of providing a service. Reimbursement may fall so low that the costs of providing that service simply are not covered. In the last 5 years, reimbursement for bone densitometry, for example, has steadily fallen to a point where it may not be sustainable in some practice settings.[13]

Keep in mind that insurance companies will typically reimburse a hospital 3 to 4 times as much as a physician's practice for the identical service. The system may say that the charge differential is related to the fact that the hospital has much higher overhead, provides charitable care, and takes care of a sicker patient mix than does the doctor's office. Although all of this is true to some extent, it is certainly true that this differential is also related to a system's clout with politicians and insurance companies who determine reimbursement.

However, a multispecialty musculoskeletal practice may find that providing a marginal service, such as DXA, has benefits to the practice, as a whole, that become obvious when you scratch below the surface. Abnormal DXA results lead to rheumatology referrals for diagnosis and treatment. Treatment may lead to infusion therapy. Osteoporosis may lead to the need for orthopedic intervention, such as kyphoplasty, fracture repair, or joint replacement. Imaging such as MRI may be required and follow-up services such as physical therapy are common. So, there builds up a certain "momentum of care," which makes the provision of DXA services integral to what we do.

FOCUS ON THE PATIENT

Medical care is becoming more and more patient/consumer focused. If a practice cannot keep up with this evolution, it really does not matter how big it is. My patients who have been seen at the Mayo Clinic routinely rave about the care they receive there. They have no idea whether the actual care they have gotten is medically superior to what they would have gotten closer to home, but Mayo's attention to patient needs and convenience is almost never off the radar screen. It makes traveling to Rochester, Minnesota in January not only a worthwhile endeavor, but downright efficient and satisfying. As we all know, the Mayo Clinic has had the wherewithal and vision to actually go to where their patients live in Arizona and Florida to make it even more convenient.

An ongoing challenge at IBJI is to find ways to make our services comfortable and convenient for our patients. Certainly, providing multiple services in one place and at one time is attractive. A readily available patient portal, federally mandated, has helped. E-mail accessibility and other simple communication devices bring us closer to our patients. We have recently begun offering urgent services every day of the week. This is a less expensive alternative to emergency room care and specifically aimed at people with bone and joint problems. This is just the kind of service that is good for the patient, good for the payer, and good for the practice. It is only one step, however, in making our services readily available. We wrestle with other access issues, such as long waits for nonurgent appointments. With 8 rheumatologists, we offer immediate appointments to all of our new patients. However, that may mean seeing someone other than the rheumatologist to whom they were originally referred, at a different location than they originally may have anticipated. It is then the patient's choice. Once a patient is in the office, what can be done to avoid prolonged waiting time? This remains a bedeviling problem for a practice where 12 physicians on a typical day at one IBJI office may see more than 400 patients with their X-rays, laboratory studies, billing and insurance questions, etc. In some cases, it will certainly involve a change in physician mindset that a patient's time is as valuable as the physician's time. Like many practices, IBJI has instituted on-line previsit registration and gradual elimination of time-consuming forms that can be handled more efficiently with electronic tools. For many of us, this frequently feels like a Sisyphean task; for every form we eliminate or shortcut we create, there is a new federally mandated consent or insurance hurdle our patients and we must overcome.

We have looked at other opportunities provided by our multispecialty model. Fracture patients are routinely referred by their orthopedist for bone densitometry and rheumatology referral. Overweight patients with osteoarthritis as well as patients with fibromyalgia and sleep disturbance can benefit from a physical therapy program that includes dietary advice and sleep evaluation. We are seeking opportunities to provide bundled care for various disease states at reduced cost with the potential for gain sharing with payers.[14]

OTHER OPTIONS

Can other models of musculoskeletal care provide the "high tech/high touch" that sits at the sweet spot of the most comfortable, convenient, and efficient care (**Box 1**)? There are pros and cons to all models, although my bias is already disclosed.

A practice involving a single practitioner certainly provides control. The corollary is that the single practitioner has to take the time to exercise that control, both administratively and, increasingly, clinically. Many solo practices have hired extenders to provide education and "routine" care. This can result in a certain amount of loss of the high-touch component that made solo practice so attractive to begin with. The additional layer of care extenders requires clinical supervision to make sure sound decisions are being made with patients who are frequently medically complex; doable, but no cake walk. Provision of ancillary services, as already mentioned, is volume dependent, so certain services may need to remain outside of the practice or are scaled to the smaller volumes of patients. Contracting terms for solo practitioners may be less attractive, on the theory that small practices can be circumvented if they do not concede more readily to payer terms. Issues such as practice coverage, sudden illness, or loss of a key employee are additional stressors. Many of these same challenges face the somewhat larger (but still small) group of 2 or 3 doctors.

Working as an employed physician for a hospital system or insurance company is certainly seen as attractive in some respects, especially by younger physicians just out, or recently out, of fellowship. The idea of a "9 to 5" job with a "guaranteed" salary sounds a lot like fellowship. There are others in the organization who do the administrative work of contracting, practice management, charges, and collections. Initially, all that the physician, her/himself, must do is simply "see the patient." Were this

Box 1
Benefits of musculoskeletal group practice
One-stop shop model
Enhanced cross-specialty consultation
Ancillary services development
Better contracting leverage
Maintains/requires ongoing physician governance
Better able to accept risk and bundling
Liability insurance economy
Supply pricing
Depth and breadth of administrative expertise
Better market access (locations, referral sources)

actually the case, it is not a bad set-up. Left unspoken is the fact that the physician is an employee with relatively little say-so in the practice management, let alone the strategic direction of the entire enterprise. Although there will be an initial salary guarantee, be assured that the guarantee will not last forever. In fact, it will last 2 or 3 years and then be readjusted to the realities of the practice (and here's the really important part) as perceived by the system management. That perception may not be shared by the involved physician and the actual facts that drive the administrative perception may not be fully shared with the doctor. The employed physician is putting a great deal of faith in a system and people that may change with each fiscal year.

Large, multispecialty group practice is yet another option. I have spoken rather glowingly about the Mayo Clinic, which is certainly the prototype of multispecialty group practice in the United States. Very few other multispecialty group practices even remotely approach the Mayo's renown and size. In most multispecialty group practices, the primary care physicians drive the group referrals and the specialists use some of their income to support primary care. There is the constant give and take between these 2 camps. If the culture is strong, the give and take becomes part of that culture and how the group does its business. If the culture is not strong, the specialists, such as rheumatologists, may perceive that they are being "penalized" to help support primary care. In addition, there is a constant tension for the resources necessary to support practice initiatives. If oncology or cardiology is a major part of the practice, it may be difficult for a rheumatologist to get her/himself heard and get the resources sought.

These comparisons obviously reflect my biases that are based on my experience not only in a focused musculoskeletal factory for the past 20 years but also in my participation in a hospital-owned, multispecialty group medical practice for almost 20 years before that. It does not mean that one cannot derive immense satisfaction and personal financial success with any of these models. Indeed, each of these models does just that on a regular basis.

GOING FORWARD

Any physician who has been involved in a strategic planning process has undoubtedly been frustrated and humbled by our inability to predict where the practice of medicine is going. There are, however, several themes that are playing out now and will remain important goals for a successful private practice (**Box 2**). The focus on the patient as the center of concern, rather than the doctor, is probably the paramount challenge.[15] Can access and communication be facilitated to the point that patients become fully engaged partners in their care? At IBJI, we are working hard to take advantage of current technologies and are looking forward to emerging technologies, such as telemedicine, to help answer simple questions quickly and triage more serious concerns in a timely manner. We are actively engaged in proactive care that anticipates patient needs, whether it is bone density evaluation on every appropriate fracture patient seen in the practice, preoperative physical therapy for total joint patients, or sleep, dietary, and psychosocial evaluation for all patients with fibromyalgia.

It is not yet entirely clear what the total impact of customized medicine and genetic analysis will have, but it is safe to say that over the next several years rheumatologists will be diagnosing disease at a much earlier stage (even before the disease develops!) and selecting medications on the basis of the genetic components of the immune dysfunction and the specific properties of the disease modifying medication.[16,17] In our lifetime, it is likely that genetic manipulation will enable physicians to stop disease

---

Box 2
The focused musculoskeletal factory in 2025

Customized appointment slots based on previous appointment experience

Thumb print/voice recognition registration

Telemedicine "walk-in clinic" for urgent advice (24/7)

Daily urgent care/routine care office hours for rheumatology

Genetic screening for at-risk patients for premorbid or early stage diagnosis

Tailored medication for specific genetic defect

Full-risk contracting for rheumatoid arthritis, psoriatic arthritis, systemic lupus erythematosus, and ankylosing spondylitis

Full-risk contracting for osteoarthritis care, including disease modifiers, and surgery

Expansion of sites of care, scope of services determined by demographic data

Rheumatology Fellowship Training

Expansion of clinical research

---

before it has occurred and to reverse disease after it has begun. More and more of this kind of diagnostic and therapeutic intervention is likely to occur in the outpatient arena, in care settings that require a multidisciplinary approach.

As already mentioned, growth of any practice remains a key goal. Without growth, a practice is at risk of being eclipsed by competitors (the "Grow or Die" maxim). The members of IBJI consider our practice a true medical center, prepared to deal with any musculoskeletal problem that presents. We are martialing our resources to provide sites of care, with appropriate specialty expertise, that are nearby and easily accessed throughout our catchment area. This means controlled but ongoing growth, not only of the services we provide, but the settings in which we provide those services. We are partnering with various payers, including Medicare, in a variety of experimental models, to provide high-value services. Some of these projects, we understand, will not be successful, but most will move the needle forward in providing better outcomes at reduced cost.

The question, going forward, is what model of practice will be best for rheumatologists, their patients, and other interested parties, such as payers. Which model will best satisfy all of these unrelenting masters? Beyond compensation, physicians are likely to do their best work and feel best about themselves when they can maintain maximum control over their practice environment. Of course, their patients must do well. A practice setting that provides comprehensive care for all musculoskeletal concerns and questions, in one place and at one time, is theoretically very attractive to patients, physicians, and payers alike. Beyond that, however, is the additional imperative that patients actually feel good about the care they receive. What will they tell their family and friends when they leave the office? What message will they send out into cyberspace? Not feeling well is difficult enough, without having additional stresses added by a practice model or philosophy that does not put the patient first.

The deciding issues will be the same for all practice models: the shift from physician focus to patient focus, the evolution from reactive to proactive care, and the best outcomes at the lowest cost (the definition of value). The focused musculoskeletal factory provides the framework to meet these challenges, while maintaining a high level of professional satisfaction for the practicing rheumatologist.

REFERENCES

1. Hochberg H. Caring, solo and small-practice doctors are becoming an endangered species. The Seattle Times 2017.
2. Rosen D. Undermining the doctor- patient relationship. Pacific Standard 2014.
3. Goold S, Lipkin M. The doctor-patient relationship. J Gen Intern Med 1999;(supp 1):526–33.
4. Herzlinger R. Market driven healthcare. Boston (MA): Addison-Wesley Publishers; 1997.
5. Kash BA, Tan D. Physician Group Practice Trends: A Comprehensive Review. Journal of Hospital and Medical Management 2016;2(1):1–8.
6. Weeks, W. Higher Healthcare Quality and Bigger Savings Found at Large Multispecialty Medical Groups, Health Affairs, Vol 29, #5, 2010.
7. Ellis K. Increasing competitive advantage in the medical office through patient satisfaction. Englewood (CO): American Coll of Medical Practice Executives; 2017.
8. Conrad DA, Noren J, Marcus-Smith M, et al. Physician compensation models in medical group practice. J Ambul Care Manag 1996;19(4):18–27.
9. Darves B. Physician compensation models: the basics, the pros and the cons. Boston(MA): NEJM Career Center; 2011.
10. Borschuk R, DeMarco C. Governance and sustaining independent physician practices. Maryland MGMA MediNews 2015.
11. Schwartz N. The doctor is in. The New York Times 2017;BU1.
12. Terry K. Questions to ask before joining a multispecialty group. Med Econ 2002;9: 124.
13. Managing in-office infusion practice. The Rheumatologist; 2012.
14. Hayes BL, Curtis JR, Laster A, et al. Osteoporosis care in the United States after declines in reimbursements for DXA. J Clin Densitom 2010;13(4):352–60.
15. Engel B, James J. Physician group practices: succeeding in bundled payments. Boston (MA): NEJM Catalyst; 2018.
16. Epstein R, Street R. The values and value of patient centered care. Ann Fam Med 2011;9(2):100–3.
17. Vogenberg F, Barash C, Pursel M. Personalized medicine (three-part series). Pharm Ther 2010;35(10):560–2, 565–7, 576.

Challenges to Practicing Pediatric Rheumatology

Nora G. Singer, MD[a,b,*], Karen Brandt Onel, MD[c]

KEYWORDS

- Pediatric rheumatology • Practice • Networks for collaboration • Critical mass
- Scholarship

KEY POINTS

- Pediatric rheumatology is an exciting and rewarding career area.
- From a lifestyle perspective, having critical mass in pediatric rheumatology divisions is important to reduce on-call frequency, and to mitigate unplanned increases in clinical work due to competing family priorities.
- Parent and patient collaboration with their providers is key to sustaining the trajectory of the field.
- Collaboration with adult rheumatology, geneticists, informaticians, and other researchers, patient groups, parent groups, professional organizations, government funders, and regulators are all key in the future success of pediatric rheumatology.

INTRODUCTION

Pediatric rheumatology is an exciting and rewarding career area. However, challenges when attracting trainees to this field include practice often occurring in smaller groups compared with general pediatrics, available positions requiring relocation, and fluctuation in graduate medical education (GME) funding resulting in uncertainty regarding training positions. From a lifestyle perspective, having critical mass in pediatric divisions is important to reduce on-call frequency and to mitigate faculty absences caused by issues surrounding family life. Compensation has historically lagged behind that of general pediatrics, especially private practice positions and behind adult rheumatology compensation. Changes in research opportunities through organized

[a] Department of Medicine, Division of Rheumatology, Case Western Reserve University School of Medicine, MetroHealth Medical Center, 2500 MetroHealth Drive, Cleveland, OH 44109, USA;
[b] Department of Pediatrics, Case Western Reserve University School of Medicine, MetroHealth Medical Center, 2500 MetroHealth Drive, Cleveland, OH 44109, USA; [c] Pediatric Rheumatology, Hospital for Special Surgery, Hospital for Special Surgery, HSS Main Campus - Main Hospital, 535 East 70th Street 5th Floor, New York, NY 10021, USA
* Corresponding author. Department of Medicine, Division of Rheumatology, Case Western Reserve University School of Medicine, The MetroHealth System, 2500 MetroHealth Drive, Cleveland, OH 44109.
E-mail address: nsinger@metrohealth.org

Rheum Dis Clin N Am 45 (2019) 67–78
https://doi.org/10.1016/j.rdc.2018.09.011
0889-857X/19/© 2018 Elsevier Inc. All rights reserved.

networks, patient and parent engagement, and the increasing recognition of pediatric rheumatologists as contributing to scholarship has heightened the profile of pediatric rheumatology in medical schools and in hospitals, as well as nationally and internationally.

Pediatric Rheumatology and the Struggle for Professional Recognition and Distinction in Academic Medicine

Pediatric rheumatology is a new specialty compared with adult rheumatology. In the United States, the original pediatric rheumatology cohort comprised a combination of pediatricians who were self-taught and/or trained by mentors interested in rehabilitation of children with chronic disease, internists with training in rheumatology, or pediatric subspecialists who shifted their practice following sabbaticals or fellowships to focus on pediatric rheumatic disease. The pediatric rheumatologists were a loosely knit group who came together first to discuss cases and then later to perform studies of nonsteroidal antiinflammatories and later methotrexate in a land mark US USSR collaborative study of methotrexate in the treatment of juvenile rheumatoid arthritis. It was not until the early 1990s that the American College of Graduate Medical Education and the American Board of Pediatrics (ABP) recognized pediatric rheumatology as a subspecialty with the first Pediatric Rheumatology Board examination being administered. In the 26years since the first examination was administered in May of 1992,[1] the professional accomplishments of pediatric rheumatologists and recognition of them has grown exponentially, but resources within pediatric rheumatology continue to be constrained. This article discusses the reasons for the lack of resources and considers potential solutions.

Financial Woes in Funding of Graduate Medical Education in Pediatric Rheumatology Compared with Adult Rheumatology and Medical Schools

Adult rheumatology has enjoyed some success in garnering funding from internal medicine departments for funding some but not all fellows with "hard money." Medicare has been the largest funder of direct GME (DGME) in the United States since 1965 when the Social Security Act created Medicare, Medicaid, and GME funding. The amount of Medicare DGME payments a teaching hospital receives is related to the share of the hospital's inpatients that are Medicare beneficiaries. All Medicare payments for DGME are paid directly to hospitals that train residents; none are made to the residents themselves. Further, in many institutions those dollars that come to the hospital via Medicare are used in part to fund the structures that support residents (indirect GME) as well as dollars to subsidize salaries (direct GME). These funding levels, based on hospital cost per resident amount and established in the 1980s, are adjusted as a percentage of the original cost but have never been recalibrated to the current costs. Further, institutions are fond of saying that they are "over cap" for the number of residency slots they have, which means they have more slots than are paid for by Medicare. For internal medicine fellowship purposes, Medicare calculates fellow salary expenses as eligible for 0.5 full-time equivalent (FTE) funding because they have exhausted the 3-year limit set by Medicare for internal medicine.[2] Thus, internal medicine–trained rheumatology fellows are often funded from a combination of clinical operating revenue (at the discretion of the chair/hospital administration), some GME dollars (at the discretion of the hospital), and endowment/philanthropic dollars and grants from organizations such as the American College of Rheumatology (ACR) and the Arthritis Foundation (AF). For rheumatology divisions that are not employees of the hospital but rather members of a faculty practice plan, dollars from infusion revenue may also subsidize fellowship training. For divisions that are wholly employed by hospitals, it is often more complex where the dollars are assigned for a hospital-based program, but, in recent years, there has been increasing recognition of so-called downstream dollars. Rheumatology divisions that garner big federal grants for the institutions and bring business to orthopedics for total joint replacement, cardiac procedures, and/or surgery caused by comorbidities as well as dollars to radiology and pharmacy are more likely to be able to negotiate strong infrastructure support, including fellowship slots, be it from their universities, medical schools, or hospitals.

Additional challenges to pediatric rheumatology training, above and beyond those mentioned, include the time and funding stream specific for pediatric GME. A requirement for funding of GME by Medicare is that the fellowship training that was a subspecialty had to be a member of the American Board of Medical Specialties (ABMS). In 1980, Earl Brewer[3] submitted an application to the ABP and that application was eventually accepted in 1990 when pediatric rheumatology joined the ABMS. Joining the ABMS was mandatory to fund fellows under the Children's Health Insurance Plan (CHIP). CHIP was the fix for improving health coverage for children and teenagers with chronic health conditions when the Clinton health care reform failed. Introduced by Ted Kennedy and Orrin Hatch with Hilary Clinton's support, it was enacted as Title XXI of the Social Security Act of 1997.[3,4] Funded by both states and the federal government, states have wide latitude in the administration of these funds. Pediatric GME is funded in part by CHIP. Until 2018, CHIP was to be renewed every 7 years and has frequently been subject to continuing resolution rather than as a budget line item. In 2017, there was a continuing resolution to fund CHIP. However, many states nearly ran out of funds before passing CHIP, which is now funded until 2027 (2017–2027). The uncertainty of CHIP has led to fluctuating funding for pediatric subspecialty fellows in general, including pediatric rheumatology fellows. Even within pediatrics, justification for apportionment of fellow slots within the department has to do to with inpatient volume because hospitals pay for hospital time. A field such as pediatric rheumatology, which is largely outpatient, will get little resource allocation. A section such as hematology-oncology within the same department with a similar number of patients will receive a disproportionate share of GME resources. Further, in many institutions, inpatient and outpatient services are funded within different funding streams and resources given by the hospital barring a high outpatient volume as justification for training slots.

One last complication unique to pediatric rheumatology has to do with fellowship length. Although most pediatric rheumatologist are engaged in clinical care, the ABP requires 3 years of training compared with the American Board Of Internal Medicine, which requires 2 years of training with an optional third year. Not only does this add expense to departments of pediatrics, generally unfunded by GME, it also delays trainees first job even if they are not interested in research and performed fellowship research only to meet the training requirement.

Pediatric rheumatology is a much younger specialty than adult rheumatology. The first Pediatric Rheumatology Council of the American Rheumatology Association (ARA) (which later split into the ACR and the AF) was formed in 1976 by Lawrence Shulman and Gerald Rodan, both presidents of the ARA. The first official US meeting of 59 pediatric rheumatologists (at least 2 were not from the United States) was in Park City in 1976, the proceeding of which was published in *Arthritis and Rheumatism* (now *Arthritis and Rheumatology*).[3,5] At the time of the first ABP Rheumatology Board Examination in 1992, 93 candidates took the boards and 80 were awarded a time-limited certificate. The second certifying examination was in 1994, with recertification initially required every 7 years. In contrast, adult rheumatology recertification is required every 10 years; however, since the original schedule was developed, the ABP has adapted their requirements to more similarly reflect the duration of adult rheumatology certification. Much to current dismay, the practice improvement modules that lacked an evidence base for their institution in the first place have yet to be removed from the ABP requirements as they were from the American Board of Internal Medicine requirements. Further, very few of the practice improvement modules directly address the day-to-day work that pediatric rheumatologists perform. The consequences of small training programs in clear. Although certification has existed for more than 25 years, total work force numbers are estimated to be no higher than 300 clinical full time equivalent (CFTE) in the United States, and are probably much lower.

Once the subspecialty was established, everyone wanted a pediatric rheumatologist but many pediatric departments/medical schools were reluctant to pay for an individual solely dedicated to the clinical practice of pediatric rheumatology. Except for those few pediatric rheumatologists who had/have a cash business, senior faculty salaries are virtually impossible to support from clinical practice of pediatric rheumatology alone. The first generation of pediatric-trained rheumatologists often thought that they were the "poor stepchild" of adult rheumatology, whereas perhaps the adult-trained rheumatologists who saw children, and for all intents and purposes who are regarded as pediatric rheumatologists, were able to push their departments of pediatrics to establish structures similar to those they experienced in departments of internal medicine. In the early days of pediatric rheumatology, it was common to build a division by trading service to the department/institution for the ability to pay for fellows or junior faculty. For example, Earl Brewer became head of the medical staff at Baylor in Houston in return for being able to fund fellowship slots, Donita Sullivan served on the institutional review board and took on other leadership positions in order to build her program in Ann Arbor.[3,4,6] Although it is common to take on additional responsibilities in any department, in pediatrics, where many pediatric divisions still have 3 or fewer faculty, it often means the difference between 50% or 33% of the on-call responsibility. It is rare to find an academic internal medicine division of rheumatology that is this small. The issue of critical mass is be discussed later in this article.

Pediatric Rheumatology Relative Value Unit Model and Compensation and Postfellowship

The relative value unit (RVU) model has in large part not only failed pediatric rheumatology but also failed rheumatology. The RVU model favors procedures over evaluation and management services. To sustain a private practice in pediatrics, seeing high volumes of children is required. Although less than 2% of pediatric rheumatologists are in private practice, the practice expense of the other services needed to provide family-centered, community-based coordinated care (FCCCC) have become unaffordable. Many academic medical services also view embedding those services within pediatric rheumatology as unaffordable. In contrast, embedding an occupational therapist in a hand clinic improves surgical outcomes and such clinics are often structured to be sufficiently busy as to justify the expense. In general, RVUs for rheumatology in private solo or large single subspecialty groups are higher than in academic centers, and some physicians in some venues do not accept insurance assignment. Root causes of reduced efficiencies in academic centers include, but are not limited to, the complexity of the patients and variability in clinic support staff that rarely report directly to the division chief. Most, but not all, academic departments in medicine have RVU expectations of their clinical staff. In pediatric rheumatology, RVUs are counted for practitioners who have only 0.2 CFTE and then extrapolated to project the RVUs for a full-time pediatric rheumatologist (reviewed in Ref.[7]). These metrics calculated by the Association of American Medical Colleges and the Medical Group Management Association may lack validity, may be biased by which organizations chooses to report, or may not exist at all because of numbers of individuals reporting. The RVU projections seem to penalize young clinicians who in turn may choose to leave the field or go part time. Those who remain frequently lag in promotions and rarely participate in faculty senates or similar groups that are limited to senior and often only research faculty.

In general, the RVU expectations for pediatric rheumatology are in the range of 70% of the adult RVU expectations, whereas salaries are often rank dependent. Pediatric rheumatology practices typically have fewer procedures than adult practices, resulting in lower streams of revenue, and telephone management that is time consuming and, in most venues, not able to be billed to insurers. New codes for telehealth may change that for pediatric rheumatology in the future.

In addition to generating fewer RVUs, to serve the population, pediatric rheumatologists often deploy to satellite clinics. These satellite clinics may be in their own health systems or through contracts with other systems that lack pediatric rheumatology and, therefore, contract for services on a more limited basis. When pediatric rheumatology was first founded, there was argument about whether clinicians should agree to deploy (led by Dr Earl Brewer and reported by him) or whether families needed to travel to the centers (argued by Dr John Miller and Dr Jerry Jacobs).[3,4] For divisions that lack critical mass (2.0 or fewer clinical FTE for pediatric rheumatology), this puts the burden on physicians who stay back to handle all urgent new patients, clinics at the primary site, and inpatient consultations (often unpredictable in number and almost always more time consuming than is reimbursed by insurance). These factors lead to dissatisfaction in faculty who are part of divisions that lack critical mass, and they scare away trainees who may be focused on both career and starting a family and require flexibility in work hours and days during the time when children are small. This lack of critical mass is first and foremost a lack of intellectual critical mass, which leads to decreased participation in registries and clinical trials that in turn holds back the entire field. It also diminishes resources to arrange for notable speakers and additional continuing medical education opportunities. Many sections supplement by uniting with their adult rheumatology colleagues but this may be challenging when located in a free-standing children's hospital. Pediatric departments also routinely fail to give credit or dedicated time to pediatric rheumatology for performing inpatient consultations, including teaching the residents who care for these patients and being available to referring physicians and parents (2 or more parents depending on the family). Pediatric rheumatology divisions that have a primary rheumatology service and not only a consultative service are better compensated for their time expenditure, and some department chairs have developed non–RVU-based metrics to evaluate clinical productivity. At most academic institutions, compensation is rank dependent, and promotion depends on scholarship and regional (for associate professor) and national or international (for profession) recognition for promotion to the rank of professor. For tenure, sustained funding and a prolific research or education (including educational scholarship) career is most often required at those institutions in which tenure still confers privileges not afforded to other faculty. Most, but not all, pediatric departments have both tenured and nontenured faculty; tenured faculty are traditionally entitled to take sabbatical leave, whereas nontenured faculty may do so at the discretion of the department chair. Practically speaking, it is difficult for anyone with a substantial patient load to be away for more than 4 to 6 months because of the critical mass issue and the need for coverage by others.

The Increase of Health Maintenance Organizations (the Role of Health and Malpractice Insurers) and the Issue of Transition from Pediatric Rheumatology to Adult Rheumatology

In the early 1990s, health maintenance organizations (narrow network products) began to increasingly refer children to adult rheumatologists if a pediatric rheumatologist was not in the network. There were outcries from pediatric rheumatology that children are not little adults and efforts, on the part of both the American Academy of Pediatrics (AAP) and the ACR representing their own membership interests, lobbied Capitol Hill for endorsement of pediatric rheumatologists as the physicians who should care for children. As policy, this was largely successful, but it was time and resource consuming for pediatric rheumatology to be recognized in its own right. Most, but not all, pediatric rheumatologists are in academic practice; those few individuals in private practice bore the largest share of advocating payment to pediatric rheumatology. These clinicians in adult private practice now frequently decline to see patients less than 18 years of age not only for the reasons discussed later but also because of concerns that, if there is a malpractice claim, insurers will regard it as out of their scope of practice and leave them exposed.

Many adult rheumatologists still think they are ill equipped to deal with childhood and pubertal issues and often are uninterested in seeing children less than 16 years of age. Historically, adult rheumatologists observed that, when transfer occurred from pediatrics to adult rheumatology, it was much more time consuming than having a new adult patient. The complexity of adults with pediatric-onset disease cannot be minimized in that children with systemic lupus erythematosus, juvenile dermatomyositis, and sometimes juvenile idiopathic arthritis have more damage than adults with similar length of disease. Young adults with a range of disabilities lack the independence and maturity of young adults without disease for both practical and emotional reasons. Frequently, the complexity of medical issues encouraged prolonged assistance by parents in dealing with appointments, medications, and insurance. Adult rheumatologists were not routinely inclined to provide care to these young adults and their families at the level of time and attention required of providers during the pediatric years. The Bureau of Maternal and Child Health program did, and continues in some states to fund a social worker and some physical and occupational therapy services within pediatric rheumatology in order to provide FCCCC. However, fee-for-service insurers, such as Blue Cross Blue Shield, failed to see the potential cost savings and declined to participate in subsidizing these services in an alternative model rather than fee for service. The population health model currently being pursued in the United States looks remarkably like FCCCC.[4,8]

Fortunately for children with pediatric adult disease, a program called Got Transition (Got Transition/Center for Health Care Transition Improvement) is a cooperative agreement between the Maternal and Child Health Bureau and The National Alliance to Advance Adolescent Health. Patience White MD, MA, a rheumatologist mentioned earlier, is the codirector and has led the initial rheumatology effort in developing policies and materials for transition in general. A Robert Wood Johnson Health Policy scholar herself, she has recruited Stacey Ardoin, MD, to colead the efforts within the ACR and there is now a transition group within the Childhood Alliance for Arthritis and Rheumatology Research (CARRA; discussed later). Transition is a national topic because poor transition is associated in all pediatric chronic disease with accelerated damage, work disability or underemployment, reduced quality of life, and increased health care expense.[9,10] Transition materials for pediatric and adult rheumatologists are housed on the ACR site (https://www.rheumatology.org/Practice-Quality/Pediatric-to-Adult-Rheumatology-Care-Transition) as well as on the Got Transition site (https://www.gottransition.org/about/index.cfm#cabinet). Use of these materials is anticipated to count as quality measures in the future and they are used in many pediatric learning health networks.[8]

Despite the frustrations noted earlier, most pediatric rheumatology fellows still choose academic career paths. A notable few pediatric rheumatologists have chosen to be in private practice or to work for industry. For most of them, a combination of circumstances has led to those decisions with no dominant trend about when in careers the transition from academia to industry has occurred. Similarly, there are several pediatric rheumatologists who have worked for the US Federal Drug Administration (FDA) (for which those of us who preform clinical trials are grateful) and there are now several pediatric rheumatologists in leadership and/or scientific positions at National Institute of Arthritis and Musculoskeletal and Skin Diseases (NIAMS) and National Institute of Allergy and Infectious Diseases (NIAID) and within the intramural programs.

Pediatric Rheumatology and the National Institutes of Health

The clinical science of pediatric rheumatology in the United States beyond using aspirin to treat juvenile arthritis began with the first group of pediatric rheumatologists[3,6] and the formation of the Pediatric Collaborative Study Group (PRCSG), led by Earl Brewer, Edward Giannini, and later Dan Lovell. The history is illustrated in part 2 of a 3-part series about the history of pediatric rheumatology. With the PRCSG as anchor, the division at Cincinnati Children's Hospital Medical Center increased in number of faculty, grant funding, and national and international prominence and has continued to show leadership in pediatric rheumatology.

The basic science underpinnings of pediatric rheumatology grew out of several centers in the same era and were largely focused on the genetics and immunology of pediatric disease. Several European and US pediatric rheumatologists spent time in laboratories at the National Institutes of Health (NIH); few US rheumatologists in the early days sustained a bench research career in part because of the clinical demands on their time and not because of lack of talent. However, over time this hurt the field; adult rheumatology had large research programs funded by the NIH that brought huge revenue to medical schools in the form of payment for indirect costs. At many medical schools and hospitals, pediatric rheumatology until the late 1980s and early 1990s was largely unable to deliver comparable funding and was viewed as incapable of amassing the patient populations required for the evolving translational science. Further, because promotion in the 1980s and 1990s was based often on numbers of articles published and so-called sustained funding, which often meant successful renewal of an RO1-level award, pediatric rheumatologists often had difficulty attaining promotion, especially to professor; this was not and is not the case in adult rheumatology.

Until the 1990s, the large US trials in pediatric rheumatology (of nonsteroidal antiinflammatory drugs and methotrexate) were largely funded by pharma and led by the PRCSG based at Cincinnati Children's Hospital Medical Center. However, in the early 2000s, NIAMS funded Dr Laura Schanberg and Christy Sandborg to conduct a multicenter trial in lupus called Atherosclerosis Prevention in Pediatric Lupus Erythematosus (APPLE). In kind, drug was supplied by Pfizer. The successful conduct of this trial, despite not meeting its primary end point, showed NIAMS, NIH, the FDA, the sponsors, and the pediatric rheumatology community the feasibility of conducting investigator-initiated trials in pediatric lupus erythematosus. Biosamples were collected, stored, and dispensed, providing for subsequent bench-based analyses and translational work. Although risky on NIAMS's part to commit these funds to teams that had not previously worked together, the foresight of Dr Susana Seratte-Sztein at NIAMS, with her faith in the team and her advice to many pediatric rheumatology grant applicants new to the NIH application system, paved the way for the current generation of pediatric rheumatology scientists. Along the same line, during a time when the NIH pay line was less constrained, the NIAID funded several more basic studies by pediatric rheumatology, especially those that were immunologically based but were constrained by the NIAMS budget. While APPLE was underway, a variety of institutes at NIH were approached about providing network funding to pediatric rheumatology, much as the National Institute of Child Health and Human Development has supported the neonatal network of the National Heart, Lung, and Blood Institute has supported a variety of heart networks. Instead, the then Pediatric Rheumatology Research Network (PRRN) was encouraged to garner infrastructure support through research projects. The PRRN was the predecessor of what is now known as CARRA.

At approximately the same time as APPLE was funded, Dr Dan Kastner and his group, who were then at NIAMS, began studying monogenic diseases. It became apparent that patients seen in the pediatric rheumatology arena, whether because of arthritis or muscle disease, cytopenias, rash, fever, or by default (unclaimed by other specialties), had been phenotyped in detail by their treating pediatric rheumatologists. By inviting these patients to NIAMS and inviting the treating physicians to participate in the ongoing care and investigation of their patients' diseases, a collaboration formed between the intramural program at NIAMS and pediatric rheumatologists. These pediatric rheumatologists, who contributed to the initial publications, were largely clinicians with academic backgrounds who had performed some research even if limited to fellowship. By thanking and including pediatric rheumatologists who had referred patients and contributed as per international committee of medical journal editors (ICJME) guidelines on publications, and by seeking an ongoing collaboration, not only was the program in monogenic disease enhanced but so was the reputation of pediatric rheumatology. When a rare disease, neonatal multisystem autoinflammatory syndrome, was discovered to be in a spectrum of disorders marked by mutations in cryopyrin, (homologous to the MEFV gene; gene product marenostrin) was published in *Arthritis and Rheumatism*, adult rheumatologists took notice.[11] Even though interleukin-1 had been previously implicated in gout pathogenesis, once the role of cryopyrin and NALP3 was recognized, there was increased appreciation about how pediatric rheumatologists could contribute to the research machine.

Although basic science research performed by pediatric laboratory-based investigators, it was the translational work that was added as a public face of pediatric rheumatology during the prior decade. Publication of (1) The Trial of Early Aggressive Therapy in polyarticular Juvenile Idiopathic Arthritis (TREAT),[12] (2) a molecular signature in systemic onset juvenile idiopathic arthritis (JIA),[13] followed by (3) RAPPORT (Rilonacept in Systemic Onset JIA)[14] all moved pediatric rheumatology forward with regard to scholarship. High regard for pediatric rheumatology at NIH by program staff and study section reviewers alike; by adult rheumatologists; and especially by other pediatric rheumatologists, their departments, and their medical schools, hospitals, and universities followed. In addition, it would be remiss not to acknowledge the Pediatric and Clinical Loan Repayment Plan, which facilitated the author's career and the careers of many others through offering some relief from student loans incurred during undergraduate and medical studies. The institution, and the survival of this important program, has been championed both by the ACR and by the AF. None of this would have been possible without the support of NIAMS and the AF support of CARRA described later.

Pediatric Rheumatology and Professional Organizations (American College of Rheumatology, Arthritis Foundation, American Academy of Pediatrics) and the Growth of the Childhood Alliance for Arthritis and Rheumatology Research

In 1991 Dr Joseph Hollander became the first Chief of Rheumatology and chief of a pediatric rheumatology division to win the prestigious Presidential Gold Medal of the ACR, an award that began in 1988. In 2002, Dr Deborah Kredich won the distinguished service award, followed by Dr Carol Lindsley in 2009 and Christy Sandborg in 2013. Awarding of senior fellow awards to several pediatric rheumatology trainees further fostered a culture of inclusion of pediatric rheumatologists within the ACR. The ACR intent was for all pediatric rheumatologists to be represented at the ACR, to be engaged in the college activities, and to benefit from and contribute to the Rheumatology Research and Education Foundation, now referred to as the Rheumatology Research Foundation (RRF). More recently, pediatric rheumatologists have a special committee (the chair attends the board of director [BOD] meetings, as do other standing committee chairs), and pediatric rheumatologists sit on the BOD of both the ACR and the RRF.

The AAP also has a subcommittee of pediatric rheumatology; participation is lower than in the ACR, but it is a home for many pediatric rheumatologists. To live immersed in a pediatric department, the AAP participation is highly regarded by department chairs and others involved in pediatric department and children's hospital administration. The Society for Pediatric Research (SPR) has a subsection of immunology in which rheumatology presentations at meetings occur.

In addition, in terms of organizing for research, CARRA, an important organization that includes pediatric rheumatology members, research nurses, and study coordinators, translational PhD researchers, and now parents, has recently become independent as a 503c entity. First funded with grants from the Wasie Foundation and the AF, CARRA has grown immensely. Rather than seek funding as a network, the steering committee (of which the author was a member) was advised to seek grant funding in which they could include infrastructure support. Two of 3 grants were funded, a Grand Opportunities grant, which paid for a build of the CARRAnet registry, and a grant to develop consensus protocols. The AF has provided funding for continued infrastructure support for CARRA. More recently, a part 11 compliant database called the CARRA registry, from which natural history can be performed, has begun. Participation by Pharma meets their phase IV FDA requirement for children, which reduces their costs. Further, this combined registry allows pediatric rheumatologists insight into how sequential drugs may contribute to both outcomes and adverse events, because children are rarely on only 1 drug throughout their lifetimes and an in-house phase IV program does not allow capture of that vital information. CARRA also provides mentoring for trainees via the AMIGO program and for study coordinators and research nurses who have their own subcommittees. The opinions shared are those of the authors and not those of MetroHealth or those of the Hospital for Special Surgery. In this, pediatric rheumatology, through necessity and by nature, has become collaborative in a way that perhaps has surpassed the larger group of adult rheumatologists. However, despite this, resources still seem to be harder to come by in pediatric rheumatology divisions despite children's hospitals being avid fundraisers.

The Patients

Children have an amazing resilience, and adolescents have ways of rebelling that frequently result in noncompliance with medications. Teenage brains are immature; I often say of lupus patients that, if I can get them from age 14 to 27 years without too much damage then I have done my job. Although it is emotionally taxing to see a small child in and out of the intensive care unit, the stressors are different than when dealing with outcomes that arise from teenagers testing boundaries or experiencing subtle cognitive defects from their disease or medication that go unrecognized. For most pediatric rheumatology children, especially those with pauciarticular and polyarticular JIA, a revisit takes minimal time if everything is going well. For providers, the most stressful time in taking care of sick children is treating children with macrophage activation syndrome (MAS) or neurocognitive changes caused by lupus or primary or secondary central nervous system vasculitis. Often there is no absolutely right answer for how to proceed (lack of evidence base). At smaller centers, the authors often use our listserv and/or call colleagues across the country for advice on those who are critically ill. Usually, in adult rheumatology divisions, there are practitioners within the division who also evaluate the patient and then discuss management, and there are usually other subspecialists who have experience and input into the clinical situation.

A most stressful outpatient situation is when it is difficult to engage all the stakeholders, and the child and/or the parents may be at odds with the child or with each other, regardless of marital status. Clinic visits concerned with issues of sleep hygiene and pain, without clear objective evidence of inflammatory disease, are stressful for some, but not all, practitioners. Lack of available neurology and psychiatry providers nationwide leaves many young people with chronic pain in the rheumatologist office. The pediatric trainees routinely state that the burden of taking care of these patients makes rheumatology an untenable option for them.

Large numbers of children live below the poverty line, and the growth of Medicaid managed care and differential acceptance of Medicaid management care plans between children's hospitals and adult hospitals, or even between divisions within the same institution, keep more impoverished young adults within pediatrics, and thus further tax a strained system. Poorer pediatric departments, which already have limited social service support, are appropriately more often focused on basic necessities for these impoverished children. As children are changed from plan to plan depending on state contracts, medications and visit referrals are required and represent a nonreimbursed expense that adds little value.

It is sometimes more difficult to care for sick children when the clinician's own children are the same age. This subject is not usually discussed in pediatric rheumatology circles, but it may occur more frequently than people expect. In addition, because many pediatric trainees expect to take care of well children, clinicians in specialties such as pediatric hematology/oncology and pediatric rheumatology need to be prepared to care for sick children, although over the past 2 decades the outlook for children with childhood rheumatic disease has improved dramatically.

Parents

Parents of children with a new or worsening chronic diagnosis are often in shock, denial, and then mourning before a reset to a new normal occurs. Other team members, in addition to the physician, need to be prepared to listen and expectantly guide new families. Disease organizations such as the AF, Cure Juvenile Myositis, the Lupus Foundation of America, and the autoinflammatory alliance group have a variety of resources available to patients and their families. Adult rheumatologists do not typically become involved with the whole family in the same way that is required of pediatric rheumatologists and only rarely have to communicate with their patients' parents. However, they may need the help of parent's adult children while caring for geriatric rheumatology patients.

Box 1
Pediatric rheumatology: challenges and potential solutions

- Pediatric rheumatology has grown significantly over the past 30 years and is now a well-recognized subspecialty
- Growth has remained low secondary to the following problems:
  - Uncertain funding for fellowship
  - Research requirement leading to prolonged training
  - Limited departmental resources for faculty hires
  - Lack of intellectual and physical critical mass
- Solutions to be considered
  - Increased participation in academic pediatric programs such as SPR and the Council of Pediatric Subspecialties (COPS) to increase recognition of the importance within pediatrics
  - Continued participation in rheumatology and pediatric networks to strengthen awareness and respect for pediatric rheumatology
  - Construct clear reasons to define need for pediatric rheumatology within the larger hospital and university framework, despite low numbers of patients and procedures.
    - Diseases are intellectually interesting and ripe for study
    - Inflammatory diseases are increasing
    - Healthy children lead to healthy adults
    - Costs to health care and hospital systems to take care of patients who have been seen late in the disease process need to be decreased

---

The Decision to Become a Pediatric Rheumatologist

Gaining exposure to pediatric rheumatology is critical in deciding to become a pediatric rheumatologist. Finding a fellowship matching, if relocation is possible, is usually not problematic because approximately 50% of pediatric fellowship training slots went unfilled in 2018. Ensuring adequate dollars for training is an institutional issue for some programs. In some institutions, pediatric rheumatology exists within adult rheumatology, whereas in most institutions it is either an independent division or combined with another division. The ins and outs of those choices are more important for first jobs. Work shortages with anticipated leaves for the birth of a new child or because of personal or family illness stress small divisions more than large divisions. On-call responsibilities become important when choosing a first job. Mentorship, career and scientific, is more limited if trainees do not have established relationships with the adult rheumatology division, whereas for adult trainees the number of potential mentors in close proximity may be greater. It is the ACR/CARRA Mentoring Interest Group (AMIGO) that serves as the model for Creating Adult Rheumatology Mentorship in Academia (CARMA), which is the mentoring program that the ACR is building for adult rheumatology trainees. Workforce shortages will challenge both pediatric and adult rheumatology in the coming years, but building the foundation for close collaboration between both should result in richer and more satisfying training and practice environments.

SUMMARY

In the past 20 years, pediatric rheumatology has grown in science, experience, and organization. Although there are still challenges in the practice of, science of, and leadership in pediatric rheumatology, the value of the field is being recognized by a variety of stakeholders. Parent and patient collaboration with their providers is key to sustaining the trajectory of the field. Collaboration with adult rheumatology, geneticists, informaticians, and other researchers, patient groups, parent groups, professional organizations, government funders, and regulators are all key in future success of pediatric rheumatology (**Box 1**).

ACKNOWLEDGMENTS

The authors thank Dr Harry Gewanter and Susan LaSalvia for thoughtful discussion and input.

REFERENCES

1. Butzin D, Guerin R, Kredich D. The first certifying examination in pediatric rheumatology. J Rheumatol 1998;25(6):1187–90.
2. Wong CA, Davis JC, Asch DA, et al. Political tug-of-war and pediatric residency funding. N Engl J Med 2013;369(25):2372–4.
3. Brewer EJ. A peripatetic pediatrician's journey into pediatric rheumatology: part III. Pediatr Rheumatol Online J 2007;5:17.
4. Brewer EJ. A peripatetic pediatrician's journey into pediatric rheumatology: Part II. Pediatr Rheumatol Online J 2007;5:14.
5. Schaller JG. The history of pediatric rheumatology. Pediatr Res 2005;58(5): 997–1007.
6. Brewer EJ. A peripatetic pediatrician's journey into pediatric rheumatology. Pediatr Rheumatol Online J 2007;5:11.
7. Henrickson M. Policy challenges for the pediatric rheumatology workforce: part II. Health care system delivery and workforce supply. Pediatr Rheumatol Online J 2011;9:24.
8. Harris JG, Bingham CA, Morgan EM. Improving care delivery and outcomes in pediatric rheumatic diseases. Curr Opin Rheumatol 2016;28(2):110–6.
9. White PH, Ardoin S. Transitioning wisely: improving the connection from pediatric to adult health care. Arthritis Rheumatol 2016;68(4):789–94.
10. Chira P, Ronis T, Ardoin S, et al. Transitioning youth with rheumatic conditions: perspectives of pediatric rheumatology providers in the United States and Canada. J Rheumatol 2014;41(4):768–79.
11. Aksentijevich I, Putnam CD, Remmers EF, et al. The clinical continuum of cryopyrinopathies: novel CIAS1 mutations in North American patients and a new cryopyrin model. Arthritis Rheum 2007;56(4):1273–85.
12. Wallace CA, Giannini EH, Spalding SJ, et al. Trial of early aggressive therapy in polyarticular juvenile idiopathic arthritis. Arthritis Rheum 2012;64(6):2012–21.
13. Pascual V, Allantaz F, Arce E, et al. Role of interleukin-1 (IL-1) in the pathogenesis of systemic onset juvenile idiopathic arthritis and clinical response to IL-1 blockade. J Exp Med 2005;201(9):1479–86.
14. Ilowite NT, Prather K, Lokhnygina Y, et al. Randomized, double-blind, placebo-controlled trial of the efficacy and safety of rilonacept in the treatment of systemic juvenile idiopathic arthritis. Arthritis Rheumatol 2014;66(9):2570–9.

Clinical Trials in Rheumatology

Christine H. Lee, MD, MPH[a], Daniel J. Wallace, MD, MACR[b],*

KEYWORDS

- Clinical trials • Rheumatology • Recruitment • Private practice
- Research coordinator • Clinical investigator

KEY POINTS

- Clinical trials serve as the basis for evaluating the benefits and harms of medical interventions with the ultimate goal of establishing an evidence-based regimen that contributes to clinical decision making.
- Clinical trials investigating rheumatic diseases in particular can be quite difficult owing to the rare and heterogeneous nature of many diseases.
- Recruitment for trials can be a challenge with factors such as location, ethnicity, language barriers, and financial status playing a role.
- If done right, clinical investigation in the changing rheumatology practice environment can be particularly rewarding and offers practitioners a variety of options.

INTRODUCTION

Clinical trials serve as the basis for evaluating the benefits and harms of medical interventions (either treatments or devices) with the ultimate goal of establishing an evidence-based regimen that contributes to clinical decision making. Those involved in the field of medicine benefit greatly from clinical research because it provides a greater understanding of epidemiology and health outcomes, and the patients they treat are given opportunities to participate in such trials. A significant reason to participate in a clinical trial often include a sense of altruism in which those with a disease want to help others who share their condition, particularly with disease states that do not have adequate therapies. Access to health care is another motivator, because clinical trial participants are able to have convenient access to care at no cost.

Disclosure Statement: None.
[a] Cedars-Sinai Medical Center, 8750 Wilshire Boulevard, Suite 350, Beverly Hills, CA 90211, USA;
[b] Rheumatology Fellowship Program, Board of Governors, Cedars-Sinai Medical Center, David Geffen School of Medicine Center at UCLA, 8750 Wilshire Boulevard, Suite 350, Beverly Hills, CA 90211, USA
* Corresponding author.
E-mail address: danielwallac@gmail.com

Rheum Dis Clin N Am 45 (2019) 79–85
https://doi.org/10.1016/j.rdc.2018.09.006
0889-857X/19/© 2018 Elsevier Inc. All rights reserved.

There is a dearth of young physicians in the field of rheumatology as well as increasing clinical workloads, which limits the amount of time that can be dedicated to research. For clinician–investigators, particularly those working in solo community practices rather than large academic centers, starting an investigative site can be rather daunting. However, once established, clinical investigation can be particularly rewarding both intellectually and help to develop a closer doctor–patient relationship. Many investigators become thought leaders, and the interaction between pharmaceutical companies and the rheumatologist often improves protocols and strengthens both groups.

TYPES AND SITES FOR CLINICAL STUDIES

Not all clinical studies are trials. Other types of studies can be observational, screen for biomarkers, genetics, or retrospective chart reviews. Clinical studies in rheumatology can screen for patient recorded outcomes or new metrics.

To understand the process of performing clinical trials, one must first understand the types of trials available. Only 2% to 5% of all candidate drugs progress from phase I to phase III and achieve approval. Phase I studies assess the safety of a drug or device. This usually takes several months to complete, usually with a small number of volunteers (20–100). The study is designed to determine the effects of the drug or device on humans, including how it is absorbed, metabolized, and excreted. Side effects that occur as dosage levels are increased are examined. A dose escalation cohort design is frequently used. About 65% of experimental autoimmune drugs pass this phase of testing.[1] Phase I studies are very labor intensive. They generally involve healthy patients who understand there is no chance they would improve with the drug. It often involves a general clinical research center in a hospital or academic setting and an overnight stay (or spending 8–12 hours at the facility). Only a handful of rheumatology practices in the United States are set up to handle this type of protocol.

Phase II studies test efficacy. This phase can last from several months to 2 years, and involves up to several hundred patients. Most phase II studies are randomized trials where 1 group of patients receives the experimental drug, and a second control group receives a standard treatment or placebo. These studies are often blinded, allowing investigators to provide the pharmaceutical company and the US Food and Drug Administration (FDA) with comparative information about the relative safety and effectiveness of the new drug. About one-third of experimental drugs successfully complete both phase I and phase II studies. The majority of phase II studies are conducted by academic sites and large group rheumatology practices.

Phase III studies involve randomized and blind testing in several hundred to several thousand patients. Typically lasting 1 to 4 years, information gathered provides the pharmaceutical company and the FDA with a more thorough understanding of the drug's effectiveness, the benefits, and the range of possible adverse reactions. Oftentimes 2 to 3 doses are tested. Of drugs that enter phase III studies, 0% to 90% successfully complete this phase. At the end of this phase, a pharmaceutical company can request FDA approval for marketing the drug. Phase III trials can usually be conducted by rheumatology practices and academic sites, and may offer an open-label extension.

Phase IV studies, also known as postmarketing surveillance trials, are conducted after a drug or device has been approved for consumer sale. This phase is meant to compare a drug with other drugs already on the market, monitor a drug's long-term effectiveness and impact on a patient's quality of life, and determine the cost effectiveness of a drug therapy relative to other traditional and new therapies. This phase can result in a drug or device being taken off the market or restrictions of use could be placed on the product depending on the findings in the study. Phase IV studies often include FDA-mandated risk evaluation and mitigation strategy–derived information. A risk evaluation and mitigation strategy is a safety strategy created to monitor known or potential serious risks associated with a medicine, often required for approval of a product.

Many phase IV trials test an approved agent for a new indication. An example would be for a rheumatoid arthritis biologic to be studied for a type of improvement seen on imaging, or change in quality of life that might be added to the drug label. Also, approved agents for orphan diseases have been studied in phase IV trials. Examples of this would include adalimumab for sarcoidosis or Behçets disease. Phase IV trials can be part of an investigator-initiated new drug application, where the drug is provided to a rheumatologist who is experienced in the area, devises the protocol, and receives funding from the pharmaceutical company.

LOGISTICAL AND PHYSICAL CHALLENGES

Logistically, many questions must be answered before participating in a trial as an investigator. One must consider whether there are a sufficient number of patients available who meet the inclusion and exclusion criteria for the study. If the sample size is too small, there may be insufficient data to reliably answer the research question. In addition, sites can be eliminated from studies if one fails to recruit enough participants, so it is important to take this into consideration before committing a site to a trial. Having an adequate number of competent and experienced clinical coordinators is essential as well. In general, for clinical trial centers, the rule of thumb is 1 full-time coordinator for every 5 studies. Given the years-long length of many trials, training 2 coordinators alleviates the burden of sudden increased workload if one coordinator requires coverage for vacation, changing jobs, and parental or medical leave.

The facility itself should have enough storage space to handle supplies, as well as identify outside facility storage if needed. Given the amount of work each coordinator must dedicate to each trial, a clerk is also needed to order supplies, take inventory, collect and spin samples, express mail, and label supplies. There should be rooms with desks for medical monitors. The delivery mechanism of the research drug should be considered as well, whether it be pills, office-administered syringes, or infusions that require monitoring over extended time periods. Monitoring visits and site investigation visits are often time consuming and detailed, and coordinators need to block out time for these visits and provide an adequate, comfortable space for their guests to work in.

Many rheumatology sites are part of a consortium or network, where budgets and contracting are common for all participants. However, in many cases, it is up to the study center to negotiate a budget. This process requires a great deal of training and experience, and can be the factor that determines the feasibility of a study. Additionally, academic sites also impose an additional layer of bureaucracy that deals with contracting, granting, patent rights, ownership of data, and indemnification. These considerations can often delay their participation by many months. Institutional overheads can range from 20% to 50% and greatly increase the study budgets.

The advent of clinical research organizations to run trials for pharmaceutical companies can be cost effective for the company, but send mixed signals to the rheumatology site. This strategy inserts an additional administrative layer that can either complicate conduct of a study or allow it run more smoothly. As of this writing, 80%

of all rheumatic disease studies involve participation of clinical research organizations. Those who have rheumatologists working for the clinical research organizations are preferred by most sites.

RECRUITMENT CHALLENGES

Recruitment for trials can be a challenge and factors such as location (urban vs rural), ethnicity (whites vs minorities), language barriers, and financial status certainly play a role. When considering which patients might be appropriate or interested for a trial, one needs to be realistic and patient while remaining motivated and taking initiative. Ciurtin and colleagues[2] conducted a cross-sectional survey of rheumatology patients in London using a questionnaire to investigate their perception and willingness to participate in clinical trials. Patients with higher versus lower levels of education had significantly higher knowledge scores. They also expressed greater willingness to take part in research (87.5% vs 48.2%; $P < .001$).[2] Those who agreed to participate in research provided significantly more correct answers. Poor disease control as the primary reason to join a clinical trial correlated well with patients' previous participation in research and the lack of understanding of research principles correlated with the lack of willingness to participate in clinical trials. Gaining knowledge of the potential barriers to recruitment allows us to address what would help potential participants to gain a better understanding about clinical trials.

Recruiting a group of participants that accurately reflects the national or global burden of disease can be difficult. Pharmaceutical companies have tended to conduct trials in Western industrialized countries, limiting the amount of information available for the efficacy and safety of treatments in non-Western populations. Although more trials are now occurring in Eastern Europe and India owing to a lack of biologic-naïve patients in the West, the Middle East and North Africa region still sponsor less than 1% of global clinical trials.[3] Practicing in a heterogeneous society such as the United States should ideally lead to recruitment of a heterogeneous sample size, but this can be easier accomplished in theory than in practice.

Falasinnu and colleagues[4] conducted a systematic review of randomized controlled trials of patients with systemic lupus erythematosus and found that the representation of blacks among randomized controlled trial participants has decreased since 2006 to 2011 in the United States, which is consistent with reviews of race/ethnic representation with other disease states. More encouraging was the finding that the inclusion of Hispanics, Asians, and Native Americans has increased over time.[4] Presumably, historical acts of discrimination and marginalization in health care settings has led to a greater distrust of health systems among racial minorities and thus an underrepresentation in randomized controlled trials. Additional consideration should be taken to train individuals who cannot only successfully manage trials, but acknowledge the differences in language, culture, and social and health literacy. Information regarding clinical research should be made available in multiple languages to prevent inaccurate translation and misinterpretation.

For the investigator, reviewing one's clinic schedule a week in advance can help to identify potential eligible patients ahead of time and streamline the process of recruitment. Having a cheat sheet of inclusion and exclusion criteria for each trial on hand can be very helpful. Garnering interest in clinical research relies heavily on the doctor–patient relationship as well as publicity. Brochures mailed to the home or placed in the waiting room with a simple "Ask us about clinical trial or research participation opportunities" can be an easy way to gauge interest levels without appearing overbearing or pushy. Appeal to the patient's sense of altruism: be comfortable, assured, look patients in the eye, and be yourself. Explain where the candidate drug fits into the broad overview of their care and how it might be a viable option to what they are already doing. Depending on what phase of trial, one can explain that the agent is already on the market for drugs being tested for repositioning, and its safety has already been studied extensively. It is imperative to reinforce that patients can drop out at any time should any adverse events occur. Never try to enroll new patients at their first appointment; without baseline rapport, this request can damage their perception of their new doctor.

Frequent concerns of potential participants include drug safety and amount of time commitment. Commonly asked questions include, "How long is the visit? How much work is missed? And How often are the visits?" Compensation for time needs to be confirmed and often times negotiated with the study sponsors to ensure participants feel enough of an incentive to participate. Creating a study protocol that is user friendly and increases compliance is crucial. Having patients or coordinators fill out time-consuming, pointless, and redundant forms has no benefit and serves as a deterrent to enrollment in future trials.

In large urban centers, patients often see more than 1 rheumatologist, and knowing other community physicians can be helpful in providing a larger subset of potential trial participants as well as establish a sense of collegial rapport among physicians.

CHALLENGES WITH RHEUMATIC DISEASES

Clinical trials investigating rheumatic diseases in particular can be quite difficult owing to the rare and heterogeneous nature of many diseases. Historically, most trials focused on rheumatoid arthritis. The advent of highly effective biologic therapies and the evolution of milder disease activity over time has diminished the pool of eligible patients. As a consequence, for many trials most participants reside outside of North America. Fortunately for these studies, well-defined outcome measures, imaging, and biomarkers make it easier to quantify efficacy than for other rheumatic disorders.

Studies for spondyloarthropathies are hampered by the very slow progression of the disease, but nevertheless several new agents have been approved in the last few years as a results of very sophisticated imaging advances. Psoriasis is easy to quantitate and score and improvements can noted rapidly.

Systemic sclerosis trials often struggle with obtaining adequate patient numbers. As a result, compromises are made in terms of study entry criteria and patient management, which can complicate the interpretation of the results. Another important aspect to consider is the extremely slow progression of disease in many patients and the fact that spontaneous improvement is often observed. This finding makes it difficult to show benefits of therapy over placebo. As a result, meaningful results are more likely to be obtained by identifying and targeting patients who are most likely to progress, rather than those who remain stable over the course of a clinical trial.[5] Such cherry picking of patients can be heavily critiqued. Identifying appropriate outcome measures is also a source of debate.

Systemic lupus erythematosus clinical trials also are notoriously difficult to conduct, not necessarily because of lack of sample size, but also because of the heterogeneity of the disease. Outcome Measures in Rheumatology, a network of health professionals established to develop validated, easy-to-use outcome measurements, established the first effort to define lupus outcomes for clinical trials in 1999. It stated that a lupus study should demonstrate improvement in disease activity, damage, health-related quality of life (via patient-reported outcomes), and toxicity/adverse events (physician-/patient-reported outcome).[6] The FDA separately came out with guidelines in 2010 for systemic lupus erythematosus drug trials, which included definitions for major flares; partial clinical responses, remission, reduction in flare; and increase in time to flare. Patients were to be stratified by severity and the British Isles Lupus Assessment Group was the preferred form of disease activity index.[7]

Unfortunately since 2005, 20 systemic lupus erythematosus drugs in phase II and III trials have failed to meet their primary endpoint using the FDA guidance document.[8] Many factors contributed to these failures, including quite simply that the drug did not work or was not safe, the trial design was flawed, a poor primary outcome measure was chosen, the trial was implemented badly, poor choice of concomitant medications allowed, artificial mandated use of steroids and tapering, or incomplete assessment of systemic lupus erythematosus activity based on the Systemic Lupus Erythematosus Disease Activity Index or British Isles Lupus Assessment Group. With many rheumatic diseases, damage indices are also not ideal target endpoints given the slow progression of these diseases.

Until recently, few trials for osteoarthritis were conducted. Over the last few years, biologic agents have finally been studied for this condition. Following a patient with involvement of multiple joints can be problematic and disease progression is slow. The advent of improved imaging and use of newer biomarkers in studies that evaluate a single joint (usually the knee) have altered the landscape of this effort.

No new drugs have been approved for fibromyalgia in more than 10 years and this complicated syndrome needs to overcome barriers that deal with measuring improvement in subjective symptoms and aspects of psychosocial distress. Very little is currently being studied for this disorder.

Most osteoporosis trials are not conducted at rheumatology sites, and use large databases. Although the number of patients in the United States with anti–neutrophil cytoplasmic antibody positive vasculitis is small, the vasculitis consortiums have been unusually successful in evaluating a variety of treatment approaches.

Gout studies usually deal with prevention of attacks since they cannot be anticipated and several anti–IL-1 approaches are being studied. Other protocols concern the long-term cardiovascular safety of existing, approved therapies. Hyperuricemia independent of gout is also a topic of interest and future clinical trials will likely be directed toward analyzing whether urate-lowering therapies are warranted in hyperuricemic individuals to lower cardiovascular and renal risk, regardless of the presence of gout.

SUMMARY

Major unmet needs in the development of clinical trials for rheumatic diseases include pediatric rheumatic disease, patients with active non–organ-threatening disease whose disease can only be suppressed with too much steroid treatments and/or are intolerant of or resistant to traditional agents, and developing validated biomarkers. As clinical investigators, physicians can often gain valuable insight into drug development and offer relevant input toward the design of future studies and trials. Performing a study correctly in a timely fashion, adhering to good clinical practice, and enrolling at least the contracted number of patients all increase the chances of obtaining further studies from the sponsor. This process helps to establish that your clinical research center is reliable and can be thought of as a highly desirable center to help conduct future trials.

REFERENCES

1. Thomas DW, Burns J, Audette J, et al. Clinical development success rates 2006-2015. San Diego (CA): Biomedtracker, BIO/Bend: Amplion; 2016.

2. Ciurtin C, Leandro M, FitzClarence H, et al. Clinical trials perception in rheumatology patients: experience from a single rheumatology tertiary center. J Rheumatol 2015;42(6):988–93.
3. Al Maini M, Adelowo F, Al Saleh J, et al. The global challenges and opportunities in the practice of rheumatology: white paper by the World Forum on Rheumatic and Musculoskeletal Diseases. Clin Rheumatol 2015;34(5):819–29.
4. Falasinnu T, Chaichian Y, Bass MB, et al. The representation of gender and race/ethnic groups in randomized clinical trials of individuals with systemic lupus erythematosus. Curr Rheumatol Rep 2018;20:20.
5. Matucci-Cerinic M, Steen VD, Furst DE, et al. Clinical trials in systemic sclerosis: lessons learned and outcomes. Arthritis Res Ther 2007;9(suppl 2):S7.
6. Strand V, Gladman D, Isenberg D, et al. Outcome measures to be used in clinical trials in systemic lupus erythematosus. J Rheumatol 1999;26:490–7.
7. US Food and Drug Administration (FDA). Guidance for industry on systemic lupus erythematosus: developing medical products for treatment. US Food and Drug Administration: Guidances (Drugs); 2010.
8. Wallace DJ. The evolution of drug discovery in systemic lupus erythematosus. Nat Rev Rheumatol 2015;11:616–20.

Challenges in Having an Infusion Center

Karen Marie Mullen

KEYWORDS

- Setting up infusion centers • Infusion center expert • Infusion therapy
- Rheumatology IV

KEY POINTS

- Sustainability and growth are at the core of a successful infusion center.
- Having a successful infusion center creates continuity and improved care, increasing patient compliance in an outpatient setting.
- A positive environment for patients is of utmost importance, with attention to the variety of elements that can lead to patient comfort and overall ease of care.

INTRODUCTION

This article is a comprehensive overview that outlines the model, care, costs, and considerations necessary in having an outpatient infusion suite in a practice.[1–3] It discusses how having a successful infusion center creates continuity and improved care, and increases patient compliance in an outpatient setting. It also provides real-life assessments of the many challenges infusion centers face, including the costs associated with establishing a center, as well as the financial and clinical impacts on practices.

To that end, this article cover how to create a positive environment for patients, with attention to the variety of elements that can lead to patient comfort and overall ease of care. From a practice standpoint, it provides a comprehensive list of specialty infusions and indications that are available, as well as the 7 options available to procure the medications necessary to run an infusion center.

There are many complexities that must be understood when considering adding an infusion center to a practice, including strategies insurance companies use to control costs, and the variety of regulations and requirements that must be met. This article provides an overview for such an analysis.

Sustainability and growth are also at the core of a successful center. Tis article discusses best practices for accepting outside referrals and the gaps that exist. It

Disclosure: None.
NewView Medical Consulting, LLC, Santa Clarita, CA 91387, USA
E-mail address: Karen@newviewmed.com

Rheum Dis Clin N Am 45 (2019) 87–100
https://doi.org/10.1016/j.rdc.2018.09.012   rheumatic.theclinics.com

provides a step-by-step plan to create an internal process for outside referrals and how to leverage them for the practice.

Successful infusion centers also use nurse practitioners (NPs) and physician assistants (PAs) in the daily operations of the practice. Each of these professionals bring their own unique approach to patient care through their training. This article examines in detail the impact, duties, benefits, credentialing, and legal requirements of these individuals in a practice.

THE BASICS ABOUT INFUSION CENTERS

Infusion centers are highly complex endeavors that require a great deal of planning and sustained focus to operate safely, efficiently, and ultimately to be cost-effective. Some autoimmune disease conditions require the use of advanced biologic medications that may necessitate intravenous (IV) administration or intramuscular (IM) injection. Successful infusion centers are pleasant and comfortable settings, with a common goal of easing the fears of patients anticipating a new form of treatment. A thriving infusion center has patients that are cared for by a staff that is uniquely trained and experienced in all aspects of IV infusion or IM injections.

CONSIDERATIONS OF HAVING AN OUTPATIENT INFUSION SUITE IN A PRACTICE

When considering the creation of an outpatient infusion suite, there are many factors to deliberate on in the purpose behind the decision as well as the short-term and long-term impact on the practice. The following outlines these considerations.

Continuity of Patient Care

Having an outpatient infusion suite allows providers to help patients better manage and control their disease by providing a continuity of care throughout their need. This ability also improves patient compliance because medical staff can monitor patient adherence to instructions, regulate and refine appropriate dosing of medication, and oversee the general progress and response to treatment. This ability creates an opportunity to provide care to patients in an ongoing, comprehensive way.

Improved Patient Care

Patients usually prefer in-office infusion suites to alternative sites of care, which may include institutional settings, because of a lower share of cost and ease of use. This setting allows the patient a more convenient and relaxed environment to receive treatment.

The overall process of the investment should be clearly understood. The return on investment can often be fast, but not immediate. Many cash-strapped practices cannot afford the short-term investment. Setting up an infusion center requires significant up-front outlays for medical equipment, pharmaceuticals, and general operating expenses. It may take time for managed care reimbursements to start coming in, especially if this is a new line of services for the practice. Therefore, clinicians must be prepared to wait several months before it is economically viable.

To achieve outstanding patient care, a series of systems and processes must be established to coordinate workflow, scheduling, and inventory management. It is highly recommended that a dedicated staff person be given total responsibility for the infusion center as their primary role in the practice. This person's responsibility is to constantly stay in touch and track all the variables required to keep patients on schedule, authorizations updated, and inventory in stock, and to reconcile all of the elements necessary to treat infusion patients. Most importantly, this individual is responsible for ensuring that the proper paperwork and submissions are completed and filed to ensure that the practice gets paid and the patient has continuous, uninterrupted access to care.

THE IMPORTANCE OF INFUSION CENTERS IN A RHEUMATOLOGY OUTPATIENT SETTING

According to the Centers for Disease Control and Prevention (CDC), as of 2012 arthritis is the most common cause of disability in the United States. Of the 54 million adults with doctor-diagnosed arthritis, more than 23 million patients say they have trouble with their usual daily activities because of arthritis. As such, infusion centers can be beneficial to both patients and providers:

- Patients can expect to receive care in a familiar setting under the care of their usual physicians
- Physicians can expect better compliance with therapy administered in the office
- In-office infusion allows further opportunity for physicians and patients to see each other, thus improving the therapeutic relationship
- There is reason to expect that infusion centers can continue to be a source of expanded revenue and value adding for infusion practices
- Hospital-based medical infusion charges are higher than those of outpatient infusion centers, and the patient's share of cost is dramatically less in outpatient infusion centers

CHALLENGES INFUSION CENTERS FACE

Infusion centers face both financial and clinical challenges, each affecting business aspects, patient communication, and overall efficiency of a practice. Infusion centers are routinely bogged down with denied insurance claims and denied prior authorization requests, which can be problematic to the overall delivery of care. Access to costly biologics is a lofty prospect, but few patients understand how IV infusions are funded. This knowledge gap can cause a multitude of problems for both the patients and the infusion facility alike. It is important to have an in-house staff who truly understand the intricacies of the various types of insurance products, and the utilization review process is key to a successful infusion operation. In the current market, infusion facilities need to be especially shrewd when it comes to the buying and billing of biologic medications. Some financial impacts that infusion centers should be aware of, and measures that should be in place to combat against them, are discussed here (**Fig. 1**).

Infusion center managers need to ensure that they have a well-trained staff, solid auditing processes, comprehensive procedures in place, on-site financial oversight at the core level of the operation, and accountability measures put in place to track the deficiencies and potential risks posed to the operation. Some of the clinical impacts a practice should also be aware of are shown in **Fig. 2**.

Costs of Running Centers

Another important challenge centers face is the startup costs and maintenance fees of managing the center. An average price range of the standard supplies necessary to start an infusion center is shown in **Fig. 3**.

Making the Patient Comfortable

An important part of overall patient care is comfort. Patients can be under a tremendous amount of stress caused by a variety of health, emotional, and financial issues.

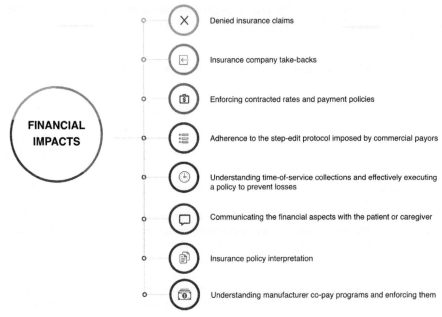

Fig. 1. Financial impacts for infusion centers.

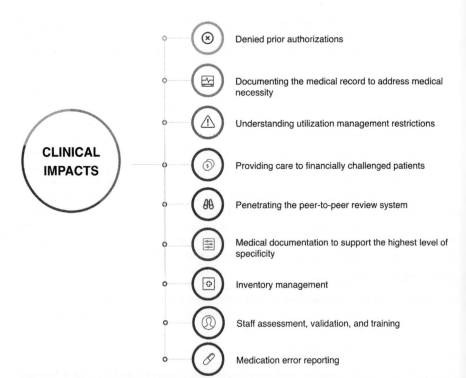

Fig. 2. Clinical impacts for infusion centers.

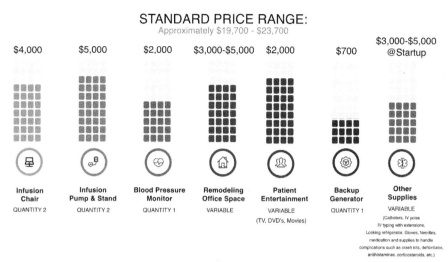

Fig. 3. Cost price ranges for startup infusion centers.

Creating a comfortable, relaxing environment can provide an outstanding patient experience. Whether planning a large-scale makeover or small touches to a facility, attention to these details can greatly improve the success of an infusion center. Some of the elements and qualities that mean the most to patients are shown in (**Fig. 4**).

Specialty Infusions and Indications

Autoimmune disease and others
There are a variety of specialty infusions available (**Fig. 5**).

OPTIONS FOR OBTAINING MEDICATION FOR COMMUNITY RHEUMATOLOGISTS

There are several options available for the procurement of necessary medications for a center. Depending on the specific situation, 1 or more of these options may be a good fit (**Fig. 6**).

- Buy and bill for the medication: the physician purchases the medication in advance and bills to insurance for reimbursement.
- Specialty pharmacy distribution: the physician submits an order to the designated specialty pharmacy, along with the clinical rationale, and the specialty pharmacy then obtains the prior authorization and dispenses the medication to the physician's office.
- Foundation programs: programs designed to assist uninsured and underinsured patients with their out-of-pocket costs on medications.
- [a]Manufacturers rebate programs: designed to assist patients with their out-of-pocket costs on name-brand biologics, strictly regulated to help patients with commercial insurance, not government plans (eg, Medicare, Medicaid, Tricare)

---

[a] Manufacturer rebate programs are an invaluable asset to both patients and physicians. Most manufacturers have created copay assistance programs to help patients manage the financial burden by covering most of the patient's drug costs. These programs provide access to the newest therapies and treatments for patients with commercial insurance who would otherwise not have access to these important medications because of the complicated manufacturing process and the high cost involved.

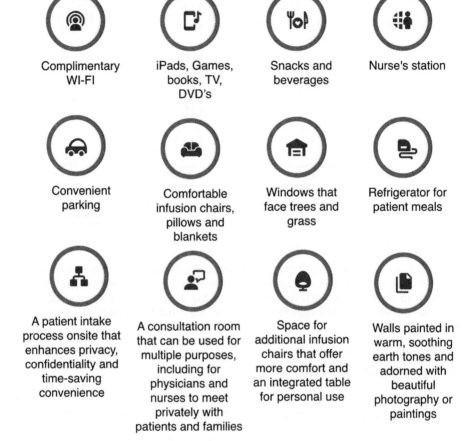

Fig. 4. Patient comfort.

- Health maintenance organizations (HMOs): providers can partner with an HMO to provide the administration of the drug and the HMO facilitates the dispensing of the drug to the site of care.
- Alternative Site of care: providers can select a designated site of care, sponsored by the drug manufacturers, infusion referral agencies, or site-of-care management companies.
- Infusion management companies: designed to partner with physicians to manage the entire infusion operation.

FAIL-FIRST REQUIREMENTS
The Impact of the Often-Overlooked Step Therapy

Step therapy, also known as a fail-first policy, is used by health insurance plans as a way to control costs. This cost-management strategy requires patients to try to document failure for 1 or more preferred treatment options before pursuing another treatment option. Many times, these fail-first requirements are not part of the medication's US Food and Drug Administration (FDA) labeling and are added into the prior-authorization process by health plans based on their own internal research or financial analysis.

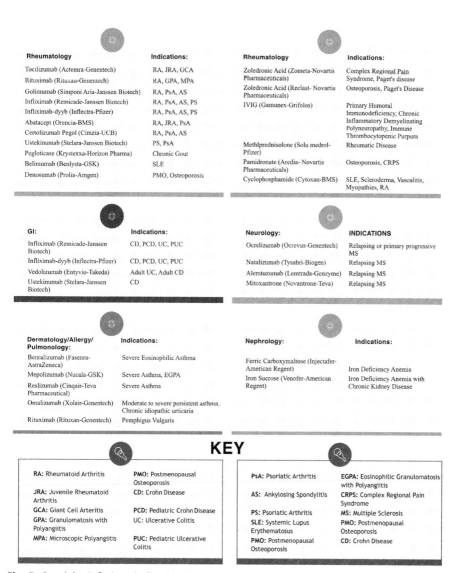

Fig. 5. Specialty infusions indications.

Step therapy requirements can often undermine a health care provider's ability to care for their patient by overruling their recommendation to pursue the prescribed treatment before trying one of the more preferred treatments required by the health plan. Step therapy is successful if the patient experiences therapeutic benefit from one of the preferred medications at a cost less than the original prescribed medications. However, many biologics, intravenous immunoglobulin, and specialty inject-ables are administered less frequently and take a long time to establish a therapeutic benefit. Patients with chronic conditions cannot afford to waste time on health plan–preferred medications if they are ineffective and the National Infusion Center Association (NICA) believes that the patients and their physicians are better equip-ped than the heath plan to select the best treatment plan. For patients with serious

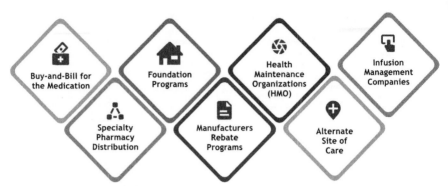

Fig. 6. Options for obtaining medication.

debilitating diseases such as rheumatoid arthritis, Crohn disease, or ulcerative colitis, every day they do not get relief is a day spent incurring long-term harm to their bodies. Delays in symptom and disease relief can result in serious complications and the need for more invasive intervention, such as surgery and hospitalization.

Denying patients access to the medications they need to improve their quality of life while wasting thousands of dollars on medications that do not work is a lose-lose situation for the patient, provider, and insurer. After all, the most cost-effective and efficacious medication is usually the one that works.

REGULATIONS AND REQUIREMENTS
What Is Necessary to Have an Infusion Center

Both the FDA's Center for Drug Evaluation and Research (CDER) and Center for Biologics Evaluation and Research (CBER) have the regulatory responsibility for therapeutic biologic products, which includes premarket review and oversight. The CDER performs an essential public health task by making sure that safe and effective drugs are available to improve the health of people in the United States. As part of the FDA, CDER regulates over-the-counter and prescription drugs, including biologic therapeutics.

The owners and operators of infusion centers must be prepared to understand and follow Centers for Medicare & Medicaid Services (CMS) rules in this area. The rules for physician supervision for infusion are more stringent in the free-standing centers and physician offices than for hospital outpatient departments in this area. Infusion centers must strictly adhere to CMS supervisor requirements. CMS requires direct supervision by physicians and this explicitly means that the physician (and not an advanced provider) must be immediately available and interruptible to provide assistance and direction throughout performance of the infusion. However, the physician does not need to be in the infusion suite throughout performance of the infusion. However, the supervising physician must be present in the office or center during the entire infusion.

ACCEPTING OUTSIDE REFERRALS IN AN OFFICE
Addressing the Gap in the Referral Process

Referrals and prior authorizations are problems for most referral coordinators in health systems throughout the United States. Having a referral management system is a unique and powerful tool for health providers to keep track of their patient referrals throughout the care continuum.

Health care is now moving toward maximizing quality and efficiency, while also minimizing cost. The entire industry is adapting to using technology as a means of streamlining administrative operations, as is evident in the widespread adoption of electronic medical record software in hospitals and clinics throughout the nation. The move toward a more unified and structured approach to documentation and caregiving is a step in the right direction.

Ultimately, the goal is to improve the overall quality of care being provided by increasing transparency, reducing operational inefficiencies, and enhancing existing processes for health care organizations both large and small.

Some alarming statistics that indicate the need for such a solution, as it relates to the topic of receiving referrals, are discussed here and shown in **Fig. 7**.

Operational inefficiencies in the medical workplace lead to bottlenecks in the care continuum. So-called dead time or unnecessarily long lead times are an inconvenience to both patients and providers alike. The 3 major factors that contribute to this are:

1. Referral workflows are inefficient and unreliable
2. Systems fail to coordinate outpatient care
3. Inefficiency leads to scheduling and payment delays[4]

To be successful at facilitating care for outside referrals, as well as to minimize the risk for liability, the receiving facility should establish an internal protocol for processing outside referrals.

The protocols shown in **Fig. 8** should be routinely offered.

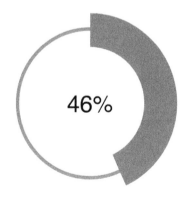

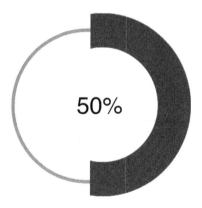

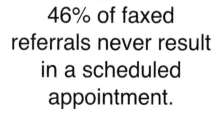

46% of faxed referrals never result in a scheduled appointment.

50% of referring physicians do not know whether their patients actually see the specialist.

Fig. 7. Referral statistics. (*Data from* Hamilton K. The true cost of poorly managed physician referrals. Available at: https://getreferralmd.com/2018/06/the-true-cost-of-poorly-managed-physician-referrals/. Accessed August 1, 2018.)

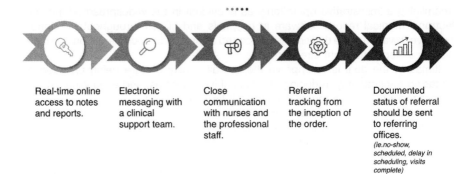

| Real-time online access to notes and reports. | Electronic messaging with a clinical support team. | Close communication with nurses and the professional staff. | Referral tracking from the inception of the order. | Documented status of referral should be sent to referring offices. *(ie.no-show, scheduled, delay in scheduling, visits complete)* |

Fig. 8. Internal protocol for processing outside referrals.

USING NURSE PRACTITIONERS AND PHYSICIAN ASSISTANTS

Successful infusion centers can leverage and use NPs and PAs in the daily operations of their practices. Each of these types of professionals bring their own unique approach to patient care through their training. NPs are trained in accordance with the nursing model, and PAs attend programs that are more in-line with the medical model, so consequently they emerge with different viewpoints and philosophies about patient care.

NPs follow a patient-centered model, whereas PAs adhere to a disease-centered model. This distinction is complex and nuanced but starts to make more sense when studying nursing or medicine at an advanced level. In the simplest terms it can be explained like this:

- The nursing model looks more holistically at patients and their outcomes, giving attention to patients' mental and emotional needs as much as their physical problems.
- The medical model places a greater emphasis on disease pathology, approaching patient care by primarily assessing the anatomy and physiologic systems that comprise the human body.

CREDENTIALING REQUIREMENTS FOR NURSE PRACTITIONERS

All NPs must complete a master's or doctoral degree program and have advanced clinical training beyond their initial professional registered nurse preparation. Didactic and clinical courses prepare nurses with specialized knowledge and clinical competency to practice in primary care, acute care, and long-term health care settings.

To be recognized as expert health care providers and ensure the highest quality of care, NPs undergo rigorous national certification, periodic peer review, and clinical outcome evaluations, and adhere to a code for ethical practices. Self-directed continued learning and professional development are also essential to maintaining clinical competency.

NPs are licensed in all states and the District of Columbia, and practice under the rules and regulations of the state in which they are licensed. They provide high-quality care in rural, urban, and suburban communities, in many types of settings, including clinics, hospitals, emergency rooms, urgent care sites, private physician or NP practices, nursing homes, schools, colleges, and public health departments. Autonomously and in collaboration with health care professionals and other individuals, NPs provide a full range of primary, acute, and specialty health care services, including:

- Ordering, performing, and interpreting diagnostic tests such as laboratory work and radiographs
- Diagnosing and treating acute and chronic conditions, such as diabetes, high blood pressure, infections, and injuries
- Prescribing medications and other treatments
- Managing patients' overall care
- Counseling
- Educating patients on disease prevention and positive health and lifestyle choices

NPs also have a variety of specialty areas and subspecialty areas (**Fig. 9**).

What sets NPs apart from other health care providers is their unique emphasis on the health and well-being of the whole person. With a focus on health promotion, disease prevention, and health education and counseling, NPs guide patients in making smarter health and lifestyle choices, which in turn can reduce patients' out-of-pocket costs.

Why Nurse Practitioners Are So Important

- Credibility: NPs are more than just health care providers; they are mentors, educators, researchers, and administrators. Their involvement in professional organizations and participation in health policy activities at the local, state, national, and international levels helps to advance the role of the NP and ensure that professional standards are maintained.
- Lower health care costs: by providing high-quality care and counseling, NPs can lower the cost of health care for patients. For example, patients who see NPs as their primary care providers often have fewer emergency room visits, shorter hospital stays, and lower medication costs.
- Patient satisfaction: with more than 870 million visits made to NPs each year, patients report an extremely high level of satisfaction with the care they receive.
- Primary care shortage solution: by offering high-quality, cost-effective, patient-centered health care, NPs provide more than 248,000 solutions to the primary care shortage currently facing the United States.[5]

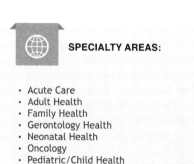

SPECIALTY AREAS:

- Acute Care
- Adult Health
- Family Health
- Gerontology Health
- Neonatal Health
- Oncology
- Pediatric/Child Health
- Psychiatric/Mental Health
- Women's Health

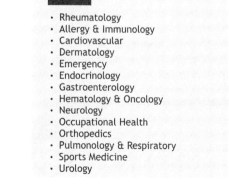

SUB-SPECIALTY AREAS:

- Rheumatology
- Allergy & Immunology
- Cardiovascular
- Dermatology
- Emergency
- Endocrinology
- Gastroenterology
- Hematology & Oncology
- Neurology
- Occupational Health
- Orthopedics
- Pulmonology & Respiratory
- Sports Medicine
- Urology

Fig. 9. NP specialty areas.

IMPACT OF PHYSICIAN ASSISTANTS

Physician assistants bring well-rounded care to the patients by offering a variety of services that treat the patient holistically as an entire person. This care can include taking time to ensure patient education is delivered, providing preventive care options and treatment, as well as managing chronic issues.

PAs' work is a great compliment to the care of the physicians and goes hand in hand with providing team care to patients. Their specific tasks may vary depending on their location, specialties, level of experience, and state laws (**Fig. 10, Box 1**).

CREDENTIALING REQUIREMENTS FOR PHYSICIAN ASSISTANTS

Physician assistants are educated at the master's degree level. According to the American Academy of Physician Assistants, there are more than 250 PA programs in the country and admission is highly competitive, requiring a bachelor's degree and completion of courses in basic and behavioral sciences as prerequisites. with them an average of more than 3000 hours of direct patient contact experience, having worked as paramedics, athletic trainers, or medical assistants, for example, PA programs are approximately 27 months (3 academic years) and include classroom instruction and more than 2000 hours of clinical rotations.

A PAs medical education and training are rigorous. The PA school curriculum is modeled on the medical school curriculum that involves both didactic and clinical education training. In the didactic phase, students take courses in basic medical sciences, behavioral sciences, and behavioral ethics.

In the clinical phase, students complete more than 2000 hours of clinical rotations in medical and surgical disciplines, including family medicine, internal medicine, obstetrics and gynecology, pediatrics, general surgery, emergency medicine, and psychiatry.[7]

LEGAL REQUIREMENTS FOR A PHYSICIAN ASSISTANT

At present, most state laws require PAs to have an agreement with a specific physician in order to practice. In 2017, the American Academy of Physician Assistants passed new policy called Optimal Team Practice, which calls for laws and regulations that remove the requirement for PAs to have an agreement with a specific physician to practice, enabling practice-level decision making about collaboration. Less than the Optimal Team Practice framework, PAs will still be legally and ethically obligated to

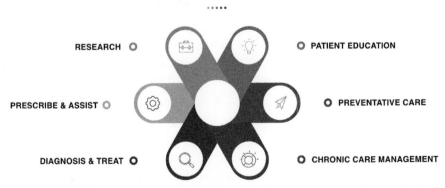

RESEARCH

PRESCRIBE & ASSIST

DIAGNOSIS & TREAT

PATIENT EDUCATION

PREVENTATIVE CARE

CHRONIC CARE MANAGEMENT

Fig. 10. PA impact.

Box 1
General duties of physician assistants

- Take medical histories
- Conduct physical examinations
- Diagnose and treat illness
- Order and interpret tests
- Develop treatment plans
- Prescribe medication
- Counsel on preventive care
- Perform procedures
- Assist in surgery
- Make rounds in hospitals and nursing homes
- Clinical research[6]

From What is a PA? American Academy of PAs. Available at: https://www.aapa.org/what-is-a-pa/. Accessed August 18, 2018.

consult with and refer patients to physicians based on the patient's condition, the standard of care, and the PA's education and experience.[8]

A GROWING PARTNERSHIP BETWEEN PHYSICIAN ASSISTANTS AND RHEUMATOLOGY

The impact of PAs in the community rheumatology setting is clearly exemplified by Christina Starks, the first community physician assist-certified (PA-C) in Hawaii to specialize in rheumatology. She is committed to practicing medicine and has a passion for helping those with gout because her father had it for more than 20 years. Christiana lives in an area of Hawaii where PA jobs are difficult to find, and, after searching for 9 months, she found a job in a rheumatology practice. She was treating a patient who was unable to walk more than 15 m (50 feet) because of gout and had softball-sized deposits of uric acid crystals. She initially prescribed the traditional form of gout medication but then remembered hearing about another novel treatment during Continuing Medical Education (CME) at the American Academy of Physician Assistants (AAPA) conference: a biologic treatment of gout that is given through IV infusions. The treatment was successful, much of the uric acid in the joints dissolved, and the patient's tophi shrank. As a result, the patient is now able to walk 2.5 km (1.5 miles). PA Starks said, "It's the only thing that can rapidly reduce the uric acid to help dissolve tophi and possibly change a patient's life." This level of training and understanding is what makes PAs an invaluable asset to community rheumatologists across the country.[9]

SUMMARY

There are many factors to consider when deciding whether an outpatient infusion center is right for a practice. A great deal of planning and decision making is required to operate a safe, efficient, and cost-effective center. From understanding the startup and operational expenses, as well as the requirements and regulations, to the financial and clinical impacts on the practice, there are many factors to consider.

A successful infusion center offers a patient-centered experience that provides a comfortable setting that eases the fears of those anticipating a new form of treatment. These centers use a staff that is trained and experienced in all aspects of IV infusion injections. These individuals play an important role in bringing their own unique approaches to patient care through their training.

ACKNOWLEDGMENTS

Research and content support, Kelly Ann Malone. Graphic and writing support, Ryan Thomas Prucker.

REFERENCES

1. Limauro MD, David L. Setting up an ambulatory infusion center in your practice. In: The American College of Gastroenterology (ACG) GI Practice Toolbox. 2018. Available at: https://gi.org/wp-content/uploads/2018/03/Setting-Up-an-Ambulatory-Infusion- Center.pdf. Accessed August 18, 2018.
2. Centers for Disease Control and Prevention. About chronic diseases. 2018. Available at: https://www.cdc.gov/chronicdisease/about/index.htm. Accessed August, 2018.
3. National Infusion Center Association. What exactly is step therapy? 2018. Available at: https://infusioncenter.org/step-therapy/. Accessed August 18, 2018.
4. Referral MD. A better way to manage your provider referral network. 2018. Available at: https://getreferralmd.com/2018/06/the-true-cost-of-poorly-managed-physician-referrals/. Accessed August 18, 2018.
5. American Association of Nurse Practitioners (AANP). Research center. 2018. Available at: https://www.aanp.org/research. Accessed August, 2018.
6. American Academy of Physician Assistants Research Center. 2018. Available at: https://www.aapa.org/. Accessed August 18, 2018.
7. American Academy of Physician Assistants Research Center. 2018. What is a physician's assistant info graphic. Available at: https://www.aapa.org/wpcontent/uploads/2018/03/What-is-a-PA-Infographic-Legal-Size_3.22_FINAL.pdf. Accessed August 18, 2018.
8. American Academy of Physician Assistants Research Center. Optimal team practice. 2018. Available at: https://www.aapa.org/advocacy central/optimal-team-practice/. Accessed August 18, 2018.
9. Walker J. Breaking ground as Hawaii's first PA in rheumatology. 2017. Available at: https://www.aapa.org/news-central/2017/10/breaking-groundhawaiis-first-pa-rheumatology/. Accessed August 18, 2018.

Challenges in Implementing Treat-to-Target Strategies in Rheumatology

Julia A. Ford, MD[a],*, Daniel H. Solomon, MD, MPH[a,b]

KEYWORDS

- Treat-to-target • Treatment strategy • Rheumatoid arthritis (RA)

KEY POINTS

- Treat-to-target (TTT), as defined in rheumatoid arthritis (RA), uses shared decision-making between physicians and patients to select a disease activity target, routinely assess disease activity, and adjust therapy accordingly to achieve and maintain the target.
- Despite evidence demonstrating improved clinical outcomes in RA using a TTT strategy, it is not widely used in rheumatology in North America.
- Access to rheumatology care, physician and patient engagement, and systems issues provide barriers to successful implementation of TTT in RA.
- Implementation of TTT in rheumatology practice requires multifaceted interventions involving the whole care team.

INTRODUCTION

Rheumatology therapeutics have grown exponentially in the last several decades with the development of targeted biologic disease-modifying antirheumatic drugs (DMARDs), as well as the routine use of combination DMARDs. Thanks to an expanded and more effective treatment arsenal, the goal of achieving low disease activity or even disease remission in certain rheumatic diseases is now feasible, and should be the expectation of both rheumatologists and patients. A natural extension of this expectation is a treatment paradigm of targeting low disease activity or clinical remission in rheumatic diseases, especially rheumatoid arthritis (RA). Treat-to-target

Disclosure Statement: Dr D.H. Solomon's work was supported by NIH-AR-072577 (VERITY). He receives salary support from research support to Brigham and Women's Hospital from Amgen, Pfizer, Abbvie, Genentech, Bristol-Myers Squibb, and CORRONA; and he receives royalties from UpToDate. Dr J.A. Ford has no disclosures.
 a Division of Rheumatology, Brigham and Women's Hospital, 60 Fenwood Road, Boston, MA 02115, USA; b Division of Pharmacoepidemiology, Brigham and Women's Hospital, 60 Fenwood Road, Boston, MA 02115, USA
* Corresponding author.
E-mail address: jrford@partners.org

(TTT) is a treatment strategy in which clinical management decisions are made with the goal of achieving and maintaining a predefined and sequentially measured target.

Outside of rheumatology, TTT approaches have been adopted in the management of chronic diseases such as diabetes and hypertension, leading to better disease outcomes.[1] However, despite a fairly strong evidence-base demonstrating the impact of TTT strategies in improving disease outcomes in RA, there is not widespread uptake of TTT in rheumatology clinics in North America. This article examines the evidence supporting use of TTT strategies, discusses barriers to implementing TTT in clinical practice, and proposes solutions and future directions for TTT implementation and research with a specific focus on RA. It briefly addresses key issues in TTT pertaining to other rheumatic diseases, including systemic lupus erythematosus (SLE), psoriatic arthritis, and gout.

TREAT-TO-TARGET PRINCIPLES AND EVIDENCE-BASE IN RHEUMATOID ARTHRITIS

The TTT model for RA is based on the core principles and recommendations as outlined by an international working group.[2,3] First, the physician and the patient should identify a disease activity target using shared decision-making. For most RA patients, the target should be clinical remission or, in some cases, low disease activity. Low disease activity may be more appropriate for patients with many comorbidities or longstanding RA. Second, disease activity should be measured regularly using a validated composite measure to assess whether patient has achieved the prespecified target. The choice of the measure is not explicitly defined but most experts agree that it should be a validated disease activity measure versus a clinician's impression (eg, disease active or doing well) and should not be a functional status score, such as the Health Assessment Questionnaire. Third, if the target has not been reached, the physician should adjust therapy at least every 3 months until the target is achieved.

Shared decision-making is a key element of the TTT approach and should be applied throughout its implementation. Shared decision-making consists of providers and patients discussing preferences and having a 2-way conversation about the risks and benefits of different treatment decisions. These decisions include the goals of treatment (ie, what is the appropriate target), whether to change treatments when disease activity is not at target or side effects may be present, and what treatment changes might be best. To achieve shared decision-making, providers must inform patients based on evidence and ensure a reasonable level of patient understanding but also they need to elicit preferences and answer questions. Through this process, patients and providers partner together to make treatment choices. Both the American College of Rheumatology (ACR)[4] and the European League Against Rheumatism (EULAR)[5] have emphasized TTT principles and shared decision-making in RA management guidelines.

Though designs differ across randomized controlled studies comparing a TTT approach with routine care in RA, they consistently demonstrate improved clinical outcomes.[6] The Tight Control of Rheumatoid Arthritis (TICORA) study[7] randomized 110 subjects in National Health Services hospitals in the United Kingdom to treatment driven by the Disease Activity Score (DAS) of 28 joints (DAS-28) with monthly assessments compared with routine care with visits every 3 months. In the TTT arm, 82% of subjects achieved EULAR good response (DAS-28 <2.4 and change in DAS-28 by >1.2) at 18 months compared with 44% in routine care arm. They also showed reduced progression of erosive disease and radiographic damage. The Computer Assisted Management in Early Rheumatoid Arthritis (CAMERA) trial[8] randomized 299 RA subjects in the Netherlands to monthly assessments and treatment adaptation via a computerized algorithm to achieve a composite target versus routine care, finding that significantly more Netherlands in the targeted control arm (35%) achieved DAS-28 remission compared with the control arm (14%) at 2 years. Fransen and colleagues[9] randomized rheumatology clinics in the Netherlands to a TTT approach to care using DAS-28 (12 clinics, 205 subjects) versus routine care (12 clinics, 179 subjects), with significantly more subjects in the TTT clinics achieving low disease activity on DAS. Symmons and colleagues[10] randomized 466 RA subjects in England to receive symptomatic care (home visits every 4 months aimed at symptom control) or aggressive care (hospital visits at least every 4 months with algorithm-based treatment changes to control both clinical and laboratory evidence of inflammation). Although both groups had similar health assessment questionnaire (HAQ) scores at 36 months of follow-up, the TTT group enjoyed better physician global assessment scores.

Although the available evidence does support improved clinical outcomes with TTT compared with routine care, the precise treatment strategy to reach a target is not clear. Several treatment target trials have compared different therapeutic strategies to reach a specified target. The FIN-RACo trial[11] randomized 195 early RA subjects in Finland to treatment with combination therapy (sulfasalazine, methotrexate, hydroxychloroquine, and prednisolone) or single DMARD therapy with a target of ACR remission at 1 year. Of subjects treated with combination therapy, 38% achieved the target versus 17% of subjects on DMARD monotherapy, which was a significant difference, and no increase in adverse events was observed in the combination therapy group. In the BeSt trial,[12] 508 subjects in the Netherlands were randomized into 4 different treatment strategies (sequential DMARD monotherapy, step-up combination therapy, initial combination therapy with high-dose prednisone, or initial combination therapy with infliximab) and treated to the target of low disease activity on DAS-44. At 2 years, significantly more subjects treated with initial combination therapy that included either prednisone or infliximab achieved low disease activity compared with patients treated initially with monotherapy. Saunders and colleagues[13] randomized 96 RA subjects in the United Kingdom to receive step-up therapy (initiating sulfasalazine, followed by methotrexate, and subsequently hydroxychloroquine) or triple therapy at onset and treated to the target of remission per DAS-28. At 1 year, both groups achieved similar percentages of subjects in remission (45% in step-up therapy group and 33% in parallel triple therapy group). As the aforementioned studies illustrate, there is not a single agreed-on treatment strategy to achieve low disease activity or clinical remission in RA.

BARRIERS TO IMPLEMENTATION OF TREAT-TO-TARGET
Access to Care

A major challenge to more widespread implementation of TTT in clinical practice is access to rheumatology subspecialty care. A systematic review of observational studies of patients with early and established RA reported that, even after publication of ACR guidelines supporting universal DMARD use in active RA, only 30% to 73% of RA patients in administrative or population-based studies (who were not necessarily under the care of a rheumatologist) were prescribed a DMARD. DMARD use in studies of subjects in RA-specific cohorts or registries (who received rheumatology subspecialty care) ranged from 73% to 100%.[14] Furthermore, in a study examining data from the National Ambulatory Medical Care Survey, only 47% of visits with a diagnosis code for RA had an associated DMARD prescription, with a visit to a rheumatologist doubling the likelihood of being prescribed a DMARD.[15]

That DMARD use is more prevalent in RA patients under the care of a rheumatologist is not surprising. Primary care physicians and other nonrheumatologists are generally not comfortable with treating RA. A survey of approximately 1000 primary care physicians in the United States, found that only one-third of respondents felt very comfortable managing this condition, and only 9% felt comfortable initiating a DMARD.[16] Factors contributing to this discomfort may include lack of continuing medical education on RA beyond medical school, lack of clear-cut treatment algorithms, and lack of familiarity with DMARDs, which are perceived as having dangerous side effects, particularly in medically complex patients.

Given what is known about nonrheumatologist discomfort with RA management and DMARD use, it is difficult to imagine TTT strategies being effectively implemented outside of rheumatology subspecialty care. Unfortunately, many RA patients do not have easy access to a rheumatologist, with regional disparities in the United States. An ACR membership database study found that 84% of micropolitan areas in the United States (population between 10,000 and 50,000) did not have a practicing rheumatologist.[17] Because demand for rheumatology care is anticipated to exceed supply in coming years,[18] the access to care problem will likely worsen.

Physician Factors

Despite being under the care of a rheumatologist, RA patients do not always receive treatment changes in the face of active disease. In a study of biologic-naïve RA patients in the Consortium of Rheumatology Researchers of North America (CORRONA) RA registry, approximately half of patients with moderate or high disease activity received treatment changes consistent with ACR recommendations for use of biologic and nonbiologic DMARDs over 6 to 12 months.[19]

In preparation for a randomized controlled trial of TTT implementation, the author (DHS) conducted qualitative interviews with 12 rheumatologists exploring use of TTT in their clinical practice.[20] Despite all interviewees believing they engaged in TTT, almost none truly followed a TTT strategy: only 3 of 12 regularly assessed a disease activity measure, 4 of 12 documented the treatment target in the medical record, and 1 of 12 engaged the patient in choosing the treatment target. This suggests that physicians may lack education on the core principles of TTT (particularly shared decision-making) or believe that their clinical gestalt of a patient's disease activity is equivalent or superior to a validated disease activity measure. The authors also suspect that some reluctance to buy into TTT among physicians may stem from resistance to standardization and algorithm-based care in medicine, which some physicians perceive as reducing their autonomy and devaluing their clinical expertise.

Patient Factors

Patient involvement is a crucial aspect of the TTT strategy. However, patients may be unwilling to escalate treatment if they are generally satisfied with their degree of disease control, despite not having reached the prespecified treatment target. A study of more than 6000 RA subjects found that 77% were satisfied with their RA medication regimen, even though 71% of these satisfied subjects had moderate or high disease activity according to the Patient Activity Score and 47% had moderate or high functional limitations on the HAQ score.[21] Satisfaction with degree of RA control, fear of side effects, and fear of loss of control of disease with medication changes were among reasons described by patients for unwillingness to change therapy. A qualitative study of 48 RA subjects identified the following themes regarding motivations to resist treatment regimens: fear of medications, maintaining control over health, denial of sick identity, disappointment with treatment, and feeling overwhelmed by the cognitive burden of deciding.[22] Themes associated with motivations to accept treatment included a desire to return to normal life, and a fear of future disability due to RA.

In addition to being willing to escalate therapy to achieve treatment targets, patients must also adhere to therapy for TTT to be successful. A retrospective study of RA patients using Medicare claims data, composed of 141 infliximab users, 853 etanercept users, and 1668 methotrexate users, found greater than 80% adherence (defined as number of therapy administrations or filled prescriptions divided by expected number) in 81%, 68%, and 64% of users, respectively.[23] Clearly, there are gains to be made in the area of ensuring patient adherence to prescribed therapies.

Systems Issues

Even in the scenario in which both patient and provider are motivated to pursue a TTT approach, constraints within the US health care system provide challenges to successful implementation. Visits every 1 to 3 months may be required to assess disease activity and adjust therapy, which may be difficult for patients to attend and for rheumatologists (who, as previously discussed, are in demand) to accommodate in their schedules. Furthermore, the pressure to see more patients and, therefore, shorten appointment times, particularly for follow-up visits, makes it difficult for rheumatologists and patients to engage in shared decision-making and to have meaningful conversations about changes in care. Tracking disease activity measures on a consistent basis, an essential principle of TTT, is perceived as time-consuming for busy providers and is usually not systemically incorporated into a practice's workflow. Finally, the often lengthy and involved process of obtaining insurance approval for DMARDs can result in delays in escalating therapy and, therefore, to achieving treatment targets, and may stand in the way of busy providers making necessary medication changes.

POSSIBLE SOLUTIONS TO CHALLENGES IN TREAT-TO-TARGET IMPLEMENTATION

Clearly, successful implementation of a TTT strategy in RA care faces multiple challenges. Possible solutions and strategies for mitigating these barriers are presented in **Table 1**. Improving access to RA care will be essential to more widespread uptake of TTT. The rheumatology community would benefit from expanding and improving medical education for nonrheumatologists in RA diagnosis and management, starting at the medical school level and extending into residency and continuing medical education, particularly for primary care and general practitioners who are on the front lines of care. Particularly because of the anticipated increasing demand for rheumatology care, young physicians should be recruited to the specialty and fellowship positions should be increased to train them. Midlevel providers, such as physician assistants (PAs) and nurse practitioners (NPs) with rheumatology training, should be increasingly integrated into care teams. The data support the effectiveness of these providers in caring for patients with RA. A nationwide survey of 174 midlevel providers in rheumatology showed that more than 90% felt comfortable diagnosing RA and prescribing DMARDs.[24] In a study of more than 300 RA patients cared for in practices with or without midlevel providers, patients seen in practices with NPs or PAs had lower RA disease activity.[25]

Mitigating physician, patient, and systems barriers to TTT first requires education of all involved parties regarding the rationale for such an approach. After both physicians and patients buy into the TTT approach, redesign of care delivery and practice workflows in the clinic may be required to facilitate successful implementation. The use of

Table 1
Barriers to treat-to-target implementation in rheumatology clinics and possible solutions and strategies for improvement

Barrier	Possible Solutions or Strategies
Access to Care	
Nonrheumatologists are often not comfortable initiating or managing DMARDs	Bolster medical school and CME training in RA and DMARDs
Many RA patients do not have easy access to a rheumatologist	Increase funding for rheumatology fellowship positions Integrate midlevel providers (NPs and PAs) into care teams
Physician Factors	
Lack of physician education on TTT principles	Integrate TTT in fellowship education and continuing medical education (CME) Develop learning collaboratives to encourage multidisciplinary team approach and patient engagement in TTT
Physician feels clinical gestalt is equivalent or superior to TTT	Educate practicing rheumatologists on TTT evidence base Collect disease activity measures and share across providers in a clinic site
Patient Factors	
Patients express satisfaction with disease control despite having active disease on validated measures	Educate patients on importance of optimizing disease control
Adherence to medications	Leverage pharmacist, nursing, and family support; reminder programs through automated programs (apps and SMS text)
Systems Issues	
Frequent visits for disease assessment difficult in busy practices	Use midlevel providers for follow-up visits
Documentation of disease activity measures is time-consuming	Use patient self-reported outcomes, including use of apps and mobile health tools Engage clinic staff (medical assistants) to assist in collection and recording
Time pressures impede shared decision-making	Develop patient-friendly resources that discuss different therapeutic options
Insurance issues delay changes in therapy	Lobby to reduce barriers to insurance coverage for patients with chronic disease

patient-reported outcomes (PROs), integration of technology to track disease activity, and learning collaboratives (see later discussion) are possible solutions to different aspects of this problem.

Patient-Reported Outcomes

PROs are signs or symptoms reported by the patient without the interpretation of a third party.[26] An example of PROs in RA is the Routine Assessment of Patient Index Data 3 (RAPID-3), a fairly widely used disease activity index comprised of PROs across 3 domains (physical abilities, pain, and overall health) that correlates with DAS-28 and the Clinical Disease Activity Index (CDAI), with the benefit of not requiring a formal joint count. How best to incorporate PROs into TTT approaches is an important question under investigation, particularly given the emphasis on shared decision-making and patient involvement in TTT. The Patient-Reported Outcomes Measurement Information System (PROMIS) pilot study[27] is examining the use of PROs in specific PROMIS domains (pain interference, fatigue, depression, physical function, and social function) using computer adaptive tests at clinic visits with RA patients being treated with a TTT strategy at an academic medical center. Baseline data have demonstrated the feasibility of incorporating PROs using PROMIS questionnaires into practice workflow.[27]

Smartphone Applications

Mobile health (mHealth) is a growing field that uses mobile devices, particularly smartphone applications (apps) to support health care. Creating apps to help RA patients monitor their disease activity and share that information with their providers has clear implications for TTT. The currently available apps intended for use by RA patients predominantly offer symptom tracking, and areas for improvement include educational content, user security, and functionality to connect to health care providers.[28]

Learning Collaboratives

Given that the multifaceted nature of TTT strategy requires the coordination and cooperation of health care providers (physicians, as well as nurses, medical assistants, and clinic staff) along with patients, the author (DHS) and colleagues pursued a learning collaborative approach for improving TTT implementation in RA. A learning collaborative uses a test, learn, and share approach consisting of sequenced learning sessions in which care teams (along with expert faculty) exchange information and brainstorm ideas, and action periods during which care teams test these ideas in their practices. Successful ideas and changes can be shared at other participating sites.[29] The Treat-to-target in RA: Collaboration To Improve adOption and adhereNce (TRACTION) trial[20] tested the effectiveness of such an approach to improving TTT implementation in rheumatology clinics. Eleven clinical rheumatology sites in the United States were randomized to a learning collaborative approach in the first 9 months (phase 1) or the wait-list control group. Intervention sites had 9 learning sessions involving expert faculty, and tested small changes in their practices and observed their effects, adopting helpful changes (in plan-do-study-act cycles). The primary outcome was a composite TTT implementation score determined through medical record review.

In TRACTION,[30] 5 sites (with 23 rheumatology providers) were randomized to the intervention arm and 6 sites (with 23 rheumatology providers) to the wait-list control. Among a sample of several hundred subjects with RA, the mean TTT implementation score was 11% at baseline in both arms; at the end of the 9-month study period, the mean TTT implementation score had increased to 57% in the intervention group and 25% in the wait-list control group, which was a statistically significant difference. There was no observed increase in resource utilization or adverse events in the intervention arm. Overall, TRACTION supports the use of an educational collaborative to improve TTT implementation in rheumatology clinics, a process that requires care delivery redesign and adapting practice workflows across care team members.

TREAT-TO-TARGET IN OTHER RHEUMATIC DISEASES

Spondyloarthritis

In contrast to RA, there are no randomized controlled trials comparing TTT to routine care in spondyloarthritis (including peripheral and axial spondyloarthritis and psoriatic arthritis).[31] However, international task force guidelines[32] embrace a TTT approach in spondyloarthritis with a recommended target of clinical remission and an alternative target of low disease activity, acknowledging importance of extraarticular aspects of these diseases. Potential barriers to effective implementation of TTT in spondyloarthritis are the heterogeneity of the patient population and the difficulty in capturing extraarticular manifestations, such as psoriasis, inflammatory bowel disease, and uveitis, into disease activity measures.

Systemic Lupus Erythematosus

Morbidity and mortality in SLE remain unacceptably high, therefore there is much interest in improving care processes for these patients. An international task force on TTT in SLE published a set of overarching principles and recommendations[33] that emphasized shared decision-making, multidisciplinary care, ensuring survival, prevention of organ damage, and prevention of flares. However, defining a good outcome or treatment target in a disease with such protean manifestations, and that affects different organ systems with varying degrees of severity, is challenging. Accrual of organ damage and adverse effects of therapies (particularly glucocorticoids) also confound the picture when assessing disease activity. The lupus community awaits validated definitions of a lupus low disease activity state and remission in SLE, which would be critical to implementation of TTT in this disease.[34]

Gout

Lowering serum urate levels to prevent crystallization of monosodium urate and crystal deposition in joints, resulting in gout, has long been a principle of chronic gout management. Treating to a target serum urate is currently endorsed by major rheumatology professional guidelines[35–37] with the recommendation for serum uric acid less than 6.0 mg/dL; however, the American College of Physicians guideline[38] contrasted substantially with the others, citing insufficient evidence for TTT in gout. Although there is no robust evidence base demonstrating efficacy of TTT serum urate approach in reducing gout flares, a 2017 EULAR abstract showed promising results. Doherty and colleagues[39] randomized 517 gout subjects in the United Kingdom to nurse-led care targeting serum urate less than 6.0 mg/dL versus routine general practitioner care. Subjects receiving nurse-led TTT care had significantly higher allopurinol dosages; a significantly greater percentage achieving serum urate less than 0.6 mg/dL; and, importantly, a significantly lower frequency of gout flares at the end of 2 years compared with the routine care group. More TTT strategy trials are needed in this disease.

QUESTIONS AND FUTURE DIRECTIONS

Many questions remain relating to TTT in RA and a proposed research agenda is presented in **Box 1**. A particularly interesting question is whether there is a therapeutic window of opportunity early in the course of RA during which aggressive treatment could meaningfully alter the disease trajectory and reduce chronicity or the need for long-term immunosuppression. A systematic literature review[40] of 18 cohort studies and randomized controlled trials reporting outcome data in early RA showed that prolonged symptom duration was associated with lower chance of DMARD-free

---

Box 1
Proposed research agenda for treat-to-target in rheumatoid arthritis

Basic science questions

1. Is there a window of opportunity during which aggressive treatment with TTT strategy can alter the course of RA?

Clinical questions

1. What is the most effective treatment strategy to reach a target of low disease activity or remission?
2. What is the optimal disease activity measure for TTT?
3. Is TTT associated with improved long-term outcomes, including reduced radiographic progression?
4. Is TTT associated with better extraarticular outcomes in RA, such as reduced cardiovascular risk?

Health services questions

1. How can mobile health technologies be optimized for TTT?
2. What are the economic costs of TTT versus routine care?

---

sustained remission, lending support to the idea of a window of opportunity in RA. One can imagine how a TTT approach could be highly valuable in this setting.

Another question of interest is whether TTT in RA is associated with improved clinical outcomes in extraarticular aspects of disease. There are some data[41,42] that suggest that lower disease activity is associated with reduction in cardiovascular risk but this has not been demonstrated in a randomized controlled trial.

SUMMARY

Though TTT for RA is supported by evidence and endorsed by major rheumatology professional organizations, this strategy for care has not been widely embraced in the United States. Creative solutions are needed at the individual provider and patient level, as well as at a systems level, to propagate a TTT approach. Although TTT may be a useful and feasible strategy for more common rheumatic diseases (and those that have a strong set of evidence-based targets), less common diseases without clear targets may not support such an approach.

REFERENCES

1. Solomon DH, Bitton A, Katz JN, et al. Review: treat to target in rheumatoid arthritis: fact, fiction, or hypothesis? Arthritis Rheumatol 2014;66(4):775–82.
2. Smolen JS, Aletaha D, Bijlsma JWJ, et al. Treating rheumatoid arthritis to target: recommendations of an international task force. Ann Rheum Dis 2010;69(4): 631–7.
3. Smolen JS, Breedveld FC, Burmester GR, et al. Treating rheumatoid arthritis to target: 2014 update of the recommendations of an international task force. Ann Rheum Dis 2016;75(1):3–15.
4. Singh JA, Furst DE, Bharat A, et al. 2012 update of the 2008 American College of Rheumatology recommendations for the use of disease-modifying antirheumatic drugs and biologic agents in the treatment of rheumatoid arthritis. Arthritis Care Res (Hoboken) 2012;64(5):625–39.

5. Smolen JS, Landewé R, Breedveld FC, et al. EULAR recommendations for the management of rheumatoid arthritis with synthetic and biological disease-modifying antirheumatic drugs: 2013 update. Ann Rheum Dis 2014;73(3): 492–509.

6. Schoels M, Knevel R, Aletaha D, et al. Evidence for treating rheumatoid arthritis to target: results of a systematic literature search. Ann Rheum Dis 2010;69(4): 638–43.

7. Grigor C, Capell H, Stirling A, et al. Effect of a treatment strategy of tight control for rheumatoid arthritis (the TICORA study): a single-blind randomised controlled trial. Lancet 2004;364(9430):263–9.

8. Verstappen SMM, Jacobs JWG, van der Veen MJ, et al. Intensive treatment with methotrexate in early rheumatoid arthritis: aiming for remission. Computer Assisted Management in Early Rheumatoid Arthritis (CAMERA, an open-label strategy trial). Ann Rheum Dis 2007;66(11):1443–9.

9. Fransen J, Moens HB, Speyer I, et al. Effectiveness of systematic monitoring of rheumatoid arthritis disease activity in daily practice: a multicentre, cluster randomised controlled trial. Ann Rheum Dis 2005;64(9):1294–8.

10. Symmons D, Tricker K, Roberts C, et al. The British Rheumatoid Outcome Study Group (BROSG) randomised controlled trial to compare the effectiveness and cost-effectiveness of aggressive versus symptomatic therapy in established rheumatoid arthritis. Health Technol Assess 2005;9(34). iii-iv, ix-x, 1-78. Available at: http://www.ncbi.nlm.nih.gov/pubmed/16153351. Accessed July 15, 2018.

11. Möttönen T, Hannonen P, Leirisalo-Repo M, et al. Comparison of combination therapy with single-drug therapy in early rheumatoid arthritis: a randomised trial. FIN-RACo trial group. Lancet 1999;353(9164):1568–73. Available at: http://www. ncbi.nlm.nih.gov/pubmed/10334255. Accessed July 15, 2018.

12. Goekoop-Ruiterman YPM, de Vries-Bouwstra JK, Allaart CF, et al. Clinical and radiographic outcomes of four different treatment strategies in patients with early rheumatoid arthritis (the BeSt study): a randomized, controlled trial. Arthritis Rheum 2008;58(S2):S126–35.

13. Saunders SA, Capell HA, Stirling A, et al. Triple therapy in early active rheumatoid arthritis: a randomized, single-blind, controlled trial comparing step-up and parallel treatment strategies. Arthritis Rheum 2008;58(5):1310–7.

14. Schmajuk G, Solomon DH, Yazdany J. Patterns of disease-modifying antirheumatic drug use in rheumatoid arthritis patients after 2002: a systematic review. Arthritis Care Res (Hoboken) 2013;65(12):1927–35.

15. Solomon DH, Ayanian JZ, Yelin E, et al. Use of disease-modifying medications for rheumatoid arthritis by race and ethnicity in the National Ambulatory Medical Care Survey. Arthritis Care Res (Hoboken) 2012;64(2):184–9.

16. Garneau KL, Iversen MD, Tsao H, et al. Primary care physicians' perspectives towards managing rheumatoid arthritis: room for improvement. Arthritis Res Ther 2011;13(6):R189.

17. American College of Rheumatology Committee on Rheumatology Training and Workforce Issues, FitzGerald JD, Battistone M, et al. Regional distribution of adult rheumatologists. Arthritis Rheum 2013;65(12):3017–25.

18. Deal CL, Hooker R, Harrington T, et al. The United States rheumatology workforce: supply and demand, 2005–2025. Arthritis Rheum 2007;56(3):722–9.

19. Harrold LR, Harrington JT, Curtis JR, et al. Prescribing practices in a US cohort of rheumatoid arthritis patients before and after publication of the American College of Rheumatology treatment recommendations. Arthritis Rheum 2012;64(3):630–8.

20. Solomon DH, Lee SB, Zak A, et al. Implementation of treat-to-target in rheumatoid arthritis through a Learning Collaborative: rationale and design of the TRACTION trial. Semin Arthritis Rheum 2016;46(1):81–7.
21. Wolfe F, Michaud K. Resistance of rheumatoid arthritis patients to changing therapy: discordance between disease activity and patients' treatment choices. Arthritis Rheum 2007;56(7):2135–42.
22. Shaw Y, Metes ID, Michaud K, et al. Rheumatoid arthritis patients' motivations for accepting or resisting disease-modifying antirheumatic drug treatment regimens. Arthritis Care Res (Hoboken) 2018;70(4):533–41.
23. Harley CR, Frytak JR, Tandon N. Treatment compliance and dosage administration among rheumatoid arthritis patients receiving infliximab, etanercept, or methotrexate. Am J Manag Care 2003;9(6 Suppl):S136–43. Available at: http://www.ncbi.nlm.nih.gov/pubmed/14577718. Accessed July 14, 2018.
24. Solomon DH, Bitton A, Fraenkel L, et al. Roles of nurse practitioners and physician assistants in rheumatology practices in the US. Arthritis Care Res (Hoboken) 2014;66(7):1108–13.
25. Solomon DH, Fraenkel L, Lu B, et al. Comparison of care provided in practices with nurse practitioners and physician assistants versus subspecialist physicians only: a cohort study of rheumatoid arthritis. Arthritis Care Res (Hoboken) 2015; 67(12):1664–70.
26. van Tuyl LHD, Michaud K. Patient-reported outcomes in rheumatoid arthritis. Rheum Dis Clin North Am 2016;42(2):219–37.
27. Bacalao EJ, Greene GJ, Beaumont JL, et al. Standardizing and personalizing the treat to target (T2T) approach for rheumatoid arthritis using the Patient-Reported Outcomes Measurement Information System (PROMIS): baseline findings on patient-centered treatment priorities. Clin Rheumatol 2017;36(8):1729–36.
28. Luo D, Wang P, Lu F, et al. Mobile apps for individuals with rheumatoid arthritis. J Clin Rheumatol 2018;1. https://doi.org/10.1097/RHU.0000000000000800.
29. Leape LL, Kabcenell AI, Gandhi TK, et al. Reducing adverse drug events: lessons from a breakthrough series collaborative. Jt Comm J Qual Improv 2000; 26(6):321–31. Available at: http://www.ncbi.nlm.nih.gov/pubmed/10840664. Accessed July 21, 2018.
30. Solomon DH, Losina E, Lu B, et al. Implementation of treat-to-target in rheumatoid arthritis through a learning collaborative: results of a randomized controlled trial. Arthritis Rheumatol 2017;69(7):1374–80.
31. Schoels MM, Braun J, Dougados M, et al. Treating axial and peripheral spondyloarthritis, including psoriatic arthritis, to target: results of a systematic literature search to support an international treat-to-target recommendation in spondyloarthritis. Ann Rheum Dis 2014;73(1):238–42.
32. Smolen JS, Braun J, Dougados M, et al. Treating spondyloarthritis, including ankylosing spondylitis and psoriatic arthritis, to target: recommendations of an international task force. Ann Rheum Dis 2014;73(1):6–16.
33. van Vollenhoven RF, Mosca M, Bertsias G, et al. Treat-to-target in systemic lupus erythematosus: recommendations from an international task force. Ann Rheum Dis 2014;73(6):958–67.
34. Morand EF, Mosca M. Treat to target, remission and low disease activity in SLE. Best Pract Res Clin Rheumatol 2017;31(3):342–50.
35. Khanna D, Fitzgerald JD, Khanna PP, et al. 2012 American College of Rheumatology guidelines for management of gout. Part 1: systematic nonpharmacologic and pharmacologic therapeutic approaches to hyperuricemia. Arthritis Care Res (Hoboken) 2012;64(10):1431–46.

36. Richette P, Doherty M, Pascual E, et al. 2016 updated EULAR evidence-based recommendations for the management of gout. Ann Rheum Dis 2017;76(1): 29–42.
37. Kiltz U, Smolen J, Bardin T, et al. Treat-to-target (T2T) recommendations for gout. Ann Rheum Dis 2017;76(4):632–8.
38. Qaseem A, Harris RP, Forciea MA. Clinical Guidelines Committee of the American College of Physicians. Management of acute and recurrent gout: a clinical practice guideline from the American College of Physicians. Ann Intern Med 2017; 166(1):58–68.
39. Doherty M, Jenkins W, Richardson H, et al. OP0268 Nurse-led care versus general practitioner care of people with gout: a uk community-based randomised controlled trial. In: Oral presentations, vol. 76. BMJ Publishing Group Ltd and European League Against Rheumatism; 2017. p. 167.1-167.
40. van Nies JAB, Krabben A, Schoones JW, et al. What is the evidence for the presence of a therapeutic window of opportunity in rheumatoid arthritis? A systematic literature review. Ann Rheum Dis 2014;73(5):861–70.
41. Solomon DH, Reed GW, Kremer JM, et al. Disease activity in rheumatoid arthritis and the risk of cardiovascular events. Arthritis Rheumatol 2015;67(6):1449–55.
42. Arts EE, Fransen J, Den Broeder AA, et al. Low disease activity (DAS28$\leq$3.2) reduces the risk of first cardiovascular event in rheumatoid arthritis: a time-dependent Cox regression analysis in a large cohort study. Ann Rheum Dis 2017;76(10):1693–9.

Digital Medicine in Rheumatology
Challenges and Opportunities

R. Swamy Venuturupalli, MD[a],*, Paul Sufka, MD[b],
Suleman Bhana, MD[c]

KEYWORDS

- Technology • Digital medicine • Social media • Virtual reality • Devices • Twitter
- Rheumatology

KEY POINTS

- Digital medicine is poised to revolutionize the practice of medicine and field of rheumatology.
- Social media use is gaining traction with rheumatology professionals increasingly engaging in social media for purposes of education, research dissemination, and career advancement.
- Virtual reality is gaining traction as a tool for behavioral modification, movement-based therapies, pain management, and simulation training.
- The authors highlight some of the technology tools currently available and being used in the clinic.

INTRODUCTION

Over the last 2 decades, advances in technology have had a transforming effect on everyday life. Who could have imagined that we would have instant access to a computer in our pockets, with the same processing power of a room full of computers from a couple of decades ago? Technology has influenced all walks of life including how we shop, eat, travel, and communicate.

In the same time period, medicine has made relatively modest strides in how we deliver care. We still rely on providing care to our patients in the same way that we did 3 decades ago with enormous effort and energy going into the documentation of care and increasingly less time being spent in actually providing care and counseling.

Disclosure Statement: Research support Applied VR- R.S. Venuturupalli. Cofounder of RheumJC on Twitter – P. Sufka. Cofounder of RheumJC on Twitter- S. Bhana.
[a] UCLA and Cedars Sinai Medical Center, Los Angeles, CA, USA; [b] Regions Hospital & Health-Partners, 401 Phalen Boulevard, St Paul, MN 55130, USA; [c] Crystal Run Health, 95 Crystal Run Road, Middletown, NY 10940, USA
* Corresponding author. 8750 Wilshire Boulevard, Suite 350, Beverly Hills, CA 90211.
E-mail address: drswamy@attunehealth.com

Just like technology has disrupted several industries such as the hospitality, transportation, and merchandising sectors, medicine stands to be transformed as well. This transformation will be facilitated by the digitization of the health record, which is nearly complete at this point in time. By some estimates in 2008, only 1 out of 10 US physicians was on an electronic medical record (EMR) but by 2018 only 1 out of 10 US physicians is not on an EMR system.[1] Other examples of significant infrastructure changes are that most patients are now connected to smartphones and a significant portion are engaged in social media. However, the single-most monumental change is in the attitude of the payers, who are now demanding an increase in the quality of care with demonstrably better outcomes obtained at a lower cost. A new field of digital medicine loosely defined as the field of medicine that uses digital tools to upgrade the practice of medicine to one that is high-definition and far more individualized has emerged.[2] Based on these observations, it seems that the complete incorporation of technology in the clinic is not only inevitable but also absolutely necessary to provide quality care to masses of people.

In this article, the authors highlight some of the promising technology trends and discuss future opportunities and challenges posed by these technologies. To comprehensively list or predict all of the important advances in technology that will likely transform medicine is not possible. However, based on the interests and experiences of the investigators, the authors have chosen to highlight the use of social media in rheumatology, virtual medicine in rheumatology, and some tech tools that are currently available to rheumatologists.

Section I: What Does Social Media Mean to Rheumatology?

The pace of electronic communication has increased rapidly, coinciding with the rapid adoption of the smartphone[3] and social media throughout the United States, with almost 7 in 10 Americans currently using at least one social media platform.[4]

Access to medical information has also become nearly instantaneous through the form of online journals, allowing for innovative methods of information sharing such as videos, slide shows, and other interactive media,[5] such as the visual abstract,[6] that can be more easily shared through social media by allowing readers a quick visual overview of an article.

Limited data suggest a trend toward increasing use of social media among rheumatology trainees. In 2014, a survey of rheumatology fellows attending the American College of Rheumatology annual meeting suggested that 40.9% of respondents were using social media for professional purposes.[7] Subsequently, a 2015 survey of European rheumatology fellows and basic scientists was conducted by the Emerging European League Against Rheumatism (EULAR) Network (EMEUNET), and found more substantial use of social media networks, with 68% using it for professional reasons such as professional networking, finding new resources, learning new skills, and establishing an online presence.[8]

Popular uses of Twitter in rheumatology include online journal clubs and discussions during medical meetings. The Rheumatology Journal Club on Twitter (#RheumJC),[7] established in January 2015, observed a total of 646 individuals from 36 different countries participate in 23 online journal club sessions over a 36-month period, with 86% indicating they were either satisfied or very satisfied with the experience.[9] Data from the 2016 ACR annual meeting also show significant use of social media, with about 20% out of more than 16,000 attendees active on Twitter during the meeting using the hashtag #ACR16.[10] Thus, the use of social media is not widespread amongst rheumatologists but seems to be increasing rapidly.

Professional uses of social media in rheumatology

Education Medical education tools and resources available on the web are collectively known as FOAMed (free open-access medical education)[11] and include sharing information and discussions on social media, as well as blog posts, videos, podcasts, and other interactive formats such as MOOCs (Massive Open Online Courses). The use of social media in medical education has also been shown to be valuable for medical students, patients, and physicians.[12]

For rheumatologists, the major intersection between FOAMed and social media can be found on Twitter. For example, the American College of Rheumatology (ACR) Twitter account, @ACRheum, currently manages a list of more than 1000 rheumatologists and health care professionals with an interest in rheumatology.[13]

Robust discussions of rheumatology-related topics can be found via networking directly with other rheumatologists on Twitter or by locating discussions using tools such as the Symplur Healthcare Hashtag Project,[14] which organizes ongoing Twitter conversations, communities, and events. Online journal clubs such as #RheumJC offer regular discussions of articles, allow participants an opportunity to develop their online network, and occasionally provide an opportunity to interact directly with authors.[15] Live-tweeting of curated information from medical conferences,[16] such as the ACR Annual Meeting or EULAR, allows for rapid sharing and dissemination to a global audience and invites discussion with those who are unable to attend the meeting in person.

Academic medicine and career advancement In the academic realm, the use of social media, especially Twitter, has been called "an essential tool"[17] that has the "potential to revolutionize academic medicine" given the "vast arrays of possibilities in which professionals, societies, and institutions can engage in conferences, education, research, and networking that extend far beyond traditional social network boundaries"[18] and its uses in allowing widely inclusive discussions, development of leadership influence, cross-disciplinary innovative efforts, scholarly dissemination of research, and mentorship opportunities.[17] In addition, the use of scholarly work within a social media portfolio has been recognized by institutions such as the Mayo Clinic as an important metric for consideration for promotion and tenure.[19]

Dissemination of research Social media has affected how information is disseminated, which required the development of new tools to measure the influence of online information. The most widely used tool for this measurement is the Altmetric score,[20] which gives real-time data on the quantity and quality of online attention that an article is receiving through news outlets, social media, citations, and downloads.[21,22] Publishers have developed promotional toolkits for investigators[23] and have suggested tips[24] that the investigators can improve the reach of their articles by promoting it on blogs, Twitter, news outlets, conferences, and via other tools such as Mendley.[25]

Professional networking and career enhancement Social media provides an opportunity for rheumatologists to broaden their professional network globally by using social media platforms such as Twitter to develop relationships with other physicians and professionals with similar interests. When used proactively, social media can be used as a powerful career enhancement tool, which can lead to opportunities related to employment, research collaboration and funding, and scientific publications and presentations.[26] In addition, social media has been recognized as a powerful tool for overcoming barriers to professional advancement of women physicians.[27]

Pitfalls in the use of social media

The use of social media in medicine certainly comes with potential pitfalls, including the accuracy of medical information, professionalism, impact on reputation, and privacy issues.[8,11] These issues are largely overcome through increased scrutiny of online information, such as by directly accessing the primary literature, or by educating users of social media regarding these issues with guidelines from the American Medical Association[28] or online courses such as the Social for Healthcare Certificate from Mayo Clinic and Hootsuite.[29]

Future directions of social media in rheumatology

Social media networks will continue to evolve and mature to meet the needs of users.

For example, Twitter recently increased the character limit per tweet from 140 to 280[30] and allowed users to link together related tweets into a thread.[31] Improving this constrained format, as well as linking together related tweets into a thread has resulted in an increase in physician engagement and discussion online.[32]

Because one of the most formidable challenges in modern medicine is organizing and keeping up with the vast amount of information, we have seen the emergence of the visual abstract as a way to rapidly share relevant data from articles via social media.

As we progress, we should expect more rheumatology professionals to engage in social media, while developing novel ways to meet their professional needs.

Section II: The Case of Incorporating Virtual Reality into the Rheumatology Clinic

Virtual reality (VR) is a technology that creates a sense of presence in an immersive, computer-generated, 3-dimensional (3D), interactive environment through head-mounted displays, body tracking sensors, and direct user inputs.[33] The promise of VR lies in the ability of this technology to transform a patient's experience almost instantaneously in a powerful way. Although initially used in the gaming world, VR has become increasingly recognized as a viable alternative for the management of pain, psychological conditions as well as simulation training in medicine.

In the rheumatology clinic, both acute and chronic pains are common presenting complaints. In addition, there are significant psychological overlays in patients suffering from the chronic diseases treated in rheumatology clinics. Coincident to the development of VR for pain is the current "opioid crisis" in the United States. From 1999 to 2014, drug overdose deaths nearly tripled in the United States[34] and the sale of opioid pain killers has nearly quadrupled from 1999 to 2010.[35] VR has the potential to provide a much-needed alternative to these agents and hence there has been increasing interest in studying this technology in patients with acute as well as chronic pain.

Mechanisms by which virtual reality potentially helps with pain

The power of VR-based interventions lies in the ability of lifelike VR gaming experiences to "hijack" the normal brain functioning and create a sense of disconnection with the patient's immediate surroundings (so-called distraction therapy). Distraction therapy has been used as a validated intervention for pain for several years,[36] and more recently, VR-based distraction therapy has also been validated in many clinical trials for pain.[37,38] Although the neurobiological mechanism by which VR acts on the brain remains unclear, researchers have hypothesized that VR can act as a nonpharmacologic form of analgesia that can unleash complex effects on the human body's pain modulation system.[39] One hypothesis states that VR may reduce the perception of pain through direct and indirect alterations in attention, emotion, concentration, memory, and other senses, which can change the body's pain modulation system.[40]

An illustrative study examined the effects of VR on the brain and showed that there was reduced activity in the insula and thalamus but other areas of pain circuitry did not seem to be affected.[41] The brain plays a complex role in the perception of pain and as such more research on the exact neurobiological effects of VR is needed to fully understand its role in pain reduction.

Utility of virtual reality in clinical medicine

Rheumatology patients present with both acute pain (osteoarthritis, crystal disease, rheumatoid arthritis [RA] flares) as well as chronic pain (fibromyalgia, osteoarthritis [OA], RA, SLE related pain). Several studies have shown that VR could reduce acute pain at least temporarily[37,42] although the literature on the effects of VR in chronic pain conditions is less robust. VR could have a wide range of uses in rheumatology. For example, rheumatologists often take care of patients with chronic lower back pain and the literature shows that VR simulations can enhance pain management by reducing pain perception and anxiety. Similarly, VR-based distraction therapy has shown to reduce the need for pain medication before burn dressing changes and in acute trauma care, where it could be used for patients with rheumatology presenting with acute pain. VR has already been shown to provide distraction therapy for diverse procedures such as lumbar punctures, cystoscopy, chemotherapy infusions, and blood draws in children. It would be easy to imagine rheumatology infusion patients using VR in a similar fashion. VR-based simulation has also shown significant utility in clinical training, particularly the mastery of procedural and interviewing skills. For a more comprehensive review of the literature supporting the use of VR in the medical clinic the authors direct the reader to an excellent recent clinical review.[43]

Rheumatologists often prescribe lifestyle modifications and physical therapy with varying results for a variety of conditions. VR has the potential of improving compliance with physical therapy programs by creating a fun gamelike environment. For example, in one study[44] patients with chronic low back pain and "kinesiophobia" were invited to participate in a VR-based dodgeball game environment over 3 days. The intervention was designed to improve lumbar spine flexibility by gradually increasing the levels of difficulty to achieve the game objective. Although this study did not reduce lower back pain (likely because the intervention was too short), the intervention was well tolerated and all patients had improved lumbar spine flexibility. The same group of investigators is planning a longer-term phase 2 randomized controlled trial, which will provide more definitive evidence for the use of VR gaming as a means to help patients with chronic low back pain.[44]

Several studies of VR have been conducted in fibromyalgia patients. A proof of concept study exposed patients with fibromyalgia to a VR-based exercise activity. In this study, when fibromyalgia patients were shown images of exercise in a virtual environment, functional MRI images demonstrated changes in brain areas associated with pain catastrophizing. Thus, interventions targeted toward pain catastrophizing using VR could be designed in the future to address chronic pain in fibromyalgia.[45] In another pilot study of 6 patients with fibromyalgia, VR was used as an adjunct to a cognitive behavioral therapy (CBT) program, primarily to help the patients develop relaxation and mindfulness skills. The intervention showed significant long-term benefits in these patients.[38] In another interesting study, investigators from Spain studied VR to enhance cognitive behavioral therapies to help patients with fibromyalgia. VR was used to improve the management of daily activities through the promotion of positive emotions, the so-called "positive technology." In this small study, the investigators demonstrated that VR-based intervention was helpful in reducing disability and also improved coping skills and perceived quality of life.[46]

VR also has the potential to augment physical therapy treatments and rehabilitation care that form the backbone of therapeutic intervention in the rheumatology clinic. For example, 40 athletes who underwent anterior cruciate ligament repair were exposed to a VR-based exercise regimen and showed improved joint biomechanics when compared with a non-VR control group.[47] In 32 elderly patients, VR based simulation exercise program showed improved hip muscle strength and balance compared to a non-VR control group.[48]

Taken together, these data show that VR is a promising new technology that could be used in the rheumatology clinic in a variety of different ways to improve outcomes.

Challenges in implementing virtual reality in the rheumatology clinic

Although VR is a significant technological innovation, it is in an early stage of development. Patients raise issues related to tolerability including complaints of nausea and vertigo after an immersive experience. Hence, VR in its current form is contraindicated in patients with severe vertigo. In one of the authors' (RSV) Rheumatology Clinic, VR-based distraction and mindfulness therapies have been piloted in about 20 or so patients. The authors' personal experience is that rheumatology patients are enthusiastic about this technology, they seem to tolerate the VR experience, and are very interested in the mindfulness programs. Cost has been an issue, although with the launch of standalone VR headsets such as Oculus Go,[49] the cost of VR is becoming significantly lower. In addition, companies in the medical VR field are innovating with their pricing plans. For example, some companies have subscription plans whereby access to numerous programs is available to patients, without a need to invest in the hardware.

As VR is incorporated into the rheumatology clinic, several important questions need to be answered. Firstly, we need to understand which patients will benefit the most and what particular immersive experience will help a particular patient or problem. A big question is whether the clinician can afford to take time from their clinical responsibilities to administer VR to patient or will there be the development of a new specialist, the digitalist. Brennan Spiegel, a leading VR researcher based at Cedars Sinai Hospital, believes that the solution would be a form of "VR Pharmacy."[50,51] Here "virtualists" who will be professionally trained in clinical medicine and VR technology will be able to evaluate patients to administer the correct corresponding VR prescription.[52] Lastly, the question of where and how VR will be administered needs to be answered. Will it be at the patient's home or in the clinic setting with superior equipment and controlled prescriptions or adjunctive therapies such as CBT? These are questions for the next phase of research in VR.

Section III: Top Tech Tools for Enhancing a Rheumatology Practice

Readily available hardware and software technology tools can augment the physician and patient experience to deliver more focused and high-quality care. Although certain technology tools such as ultrasound are being implemented in rheumatology practices around the world, one could argue that device cost, training time, and strain on workflow can be prohibitive to widespread adoption.[53,54] The ideal implementation of particular technology products relies on the principals of cost, time, usability, and effect on patient outcomes. Although technology holds great promise in changing the way we practice, we are still in the early stages of implementing new technologies in the clinic. This point is well illustrated in a recent study that examined the utility of fitness trackers and apps and found that there was no significant change in health outcomes for patients by the use of these apps and devices.[55]

The popularity and power of the smartphone is a driving force in the implementation of personal and portable technology in the clinic. At its core, the smartphone is a combination of a microcomputer, camera, contextual sensors, and constant internet connection for all applications. Each year, the smartphone models become increasingly more powerful. As of the end of 2017, the iPhone X processing benchmarks were equal to a 2017 Macbook Pro.[56] This unprecedented processing power could transform how the clinician patient interaction takes place. Although a comprehensive listing of portable technology in the clinic is not possible, in the following section, we highlight some of the most practical and accessible tools as of the time of this writing (June 2018) that could help rheumatologists in the care of their patients. These tools were chosen based on low entry price compared with medical device grade products, usability and design, and portability, and testing in the rheumatology clinic by one of the authors (SB). A summary of the tools and their applications is presented in **Table 1**.

Hardware tools
A variety of inexpensive hardware tools, which tend to focus on enhanced imaging techniques, can aid the diagnosis and management of a subset of rheumatic patients.

Macro lens for nailfold capillaroscopy Nailfold capillaroscopy (NC) is the most reliable way to distinguish between primary and secondary Raynaud phenomenon (RP).[4,57] NC is part of the ACR/EULAR classification for systemic sclerosis. In clinical studies 200x-magnification ophthalmoscope is typically used; however, a standard handheld ophthalmoscope only provides 2 to 3x magnification when repurposed for NC. Handheld lighted magnification devices used by dermatologists can provide 10x magnification but cost $500 or higher. Alternatively, the OlloClip Macro Pro Lens, a consumer external lens kit for iPhone can clip to the smartphone's camera and provide up to 21x optical magnification (**Fig. 1**). When combined with the smartphone's built-in digital zoom, up to 31x magnification can be achieved, as well as being able to capture pictures and live video without emersion oil or gel.

Thermal imaging Thermal imaging (TI) is a rapid, highly reproducible method of using infrared imaging to quantitate the degree of inflammation in animal models of RA.[58] Infrared imaging in RA can distinguish disease severity with a sensitivity and specificity of 96% and 92%, respectively compared with normal control.[59] TI can distinguish Raynaud temperature differences in a women's first toe with a sensitivity and specificity or 73% and 66%, respectively compared with healthy controls.[38] Other non-Raynaud vascular disorders can be assessed with TI (**Fig. 2**). Commercial grade TI cameras can be thousands of dollars per device. Alternatively, the forward-looking infrared ONE thermal imaging camera is a smartphone attachment that can be used for medical applications. This device attaches to a smartphone or tablet via the dataport and combines both a thermal camera and standard camera to composite a dual image with added detail. The manufacturer states the ability to detect temperature differences as small as 0.18°F (0.1°C) ($199 FLIR ONE).

Microscope imaging Synovial fluid microscopy is still the gold standard diagnostic modality for crystalline arthropathy.[60] Traditional image capture equipment for a tabletop microscope can exceed $1000, with added cost and complexity for captured and live streaming video. Alternatively, a mounting bracket for a smartphone can be attached to the left or right eye piece of a microscope for optical to digital image and video capture. One example is the Gosky Universal Cell Phone Adapter Mount ($24.99), which can capture still images plus video, and use digital zoom. In addition, the smartphone can stream to an external display or still use live video chat (eg, Skype or FaceTime).

Table 1
Emerging innovative tools for use in rheumatology

Device/Software	Description	Potential Use
OlloClip Macro Pro Lens (Hardware tool)	External lens kit for iPhone can clip to the smartphone camera and provide up to 21x – 31x optical magnification for nailfold capillaroscopy	Scleroderma, connective tissue disease monitoring
Forward-looking Infrared ONE Thermal Imaging Camera (Hardware tool)	Smartphone attachment that combines both a thermal camera and standard camera to composite a dual image with added detail. Could detect temperature differences as small as 0.18°F (0.1°C)	Inflammatory arthritis, CRPS, vasculitis monitoring
Gosky Universal Cell Phone Adapter Mount (Hardware tool)	Fits eyepiece of smartphone. Can be used as an alternative to traditional image capture equipment of synovial fluid microscopy	Synovial fluid analysis and other microscopy
3D4Medical Application (Software tool)	Software using 3-dimensional, real-time rendered images and video, based on MRI and CT reconstructions	Education of patients, practitioners
DAS Calc (Software tool)	Can calculate a variety of disease activity instruments such as DAS28 (3 or 4 Variable), Disease Activity Score C-Reactive Protein (DAS-CRP), Clinical Disease Activity Index (CDAI), Simple Disease Activity Index (SDAI), and Routine Assessment of Patient Index Data 3 (RAPID3)	Rheumatoid activity monitoring
Psoriasis Calc (Software tool)	Software application to calculate the PASI score	Psoriasis activity monitoring

Abbreviations: CRPS, complex regional pain syndrome; CT, computed tomography; PASI, Psoriasis Area and Severity Index.

These innovative hardware tools offer a low-cost alternative that can promote the integration of technology into rheumatology.

Software tools
There are several opportunities for the use of software tools in the medical office. Innovative software tools can assist with patient education, informing consent, improved compliance, education of trainees, and EMR workflows.

Anatomic applications Anatomy software has been ubiquitous in medical education for decades. Besides education of trainees and practicing physicians, patient education can be enhanced with medical software.[61,62] 3D4Medical is a top rated anatomy software developer for the iOS, Android, and Mac operating systems using 3D, real-time rendered images, and video, based on MRI and computed tomography reconstructions. Newly added features include augmented reality mode to overlay 3D

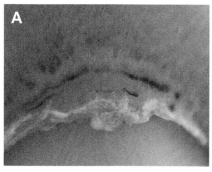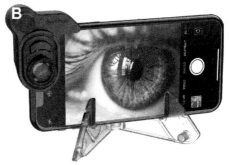

Fig. 1. (*A*) A patient with limited cutaneous systemic sclerosis, interstitial lung disease, and pulmonary hypertension. Image captured using an iPhone 7 and a 2016 OlloClip Macro Lens with 21x magnification. (*B*) Means of attachment of 2017 OlloClip to iPhone X.

reconstructions within the real world. Software from this developer is used in universities and physician offices throughout the world, with affordable costs of apps ranging from $7.99 to $59.99.

Clinical applications The Disease Activity Score 28 point joint count (DAS28) remains a ubiquitous disease activity instrument for inflammatory arthritis. There is a handful of rheumatology-dedicated EMRs that can calculate this but most multipurpose EMRs still do not contain this function. DAS Calc is an offline smartphone application for iOS devices that can calculate a variety of disease activity instruments as mentioned in **Table 1**.

Similarly, Psoriasis Calc is a free application for iOS and Android smartphones that enables quick calculation for body surface area involvement of psoriasis and has a visual guide and calculator to generate a Psoriasis Area and Severity Index score. Both of these applications are widely applicable in rheumatology practices due to the prevalence of these diseases with many of the patients encountered.

Patient applications Obesity is a common risk factor for rheumatic disease, with many patients struggling with even modest weight loss. Although there is no substitute for a regular exercise routine and formal dietary counseling, there are several smartphone applications designed to aid in weight loss. One example amongst many is Lose It! (free with premium features), a multiplatform smartphone and Web application that enables tailor-made calorie counting based on user-defined goals enhanced with gamification and a social component. Lose It! integrates with connected health devices such as fitness bands, smart watches, weight scales, and blood pressure cuffs. Fitness bands can also be used in clinical trials to gather data on the efficiency of different weight loss methods in research studies.

Chronic pain remains a leading cause of disability and it is a major contributor to health care costs, with one in every 4 Americans having suffered from pain that lasts longer than 24 hours.[63] Although this problem is extraordinarily complex in terms of long-term management, meditation and mindfulness-based stress reduction (MMBSR) has been shown to be effective in modulating through endogenous opioids.[64] In addition, MMBSR is associated with significant deactivation of regions of the default mode network, the region of the brain that is dysfunctional in chronic pain, fibromyalgia, mood, and cognitive disorders.[65] Along with several applications currently available, Calm (free with premium features) is a multiplatform app for MMBSR. Calm allows users to choose different mindfulness programs spanning 1

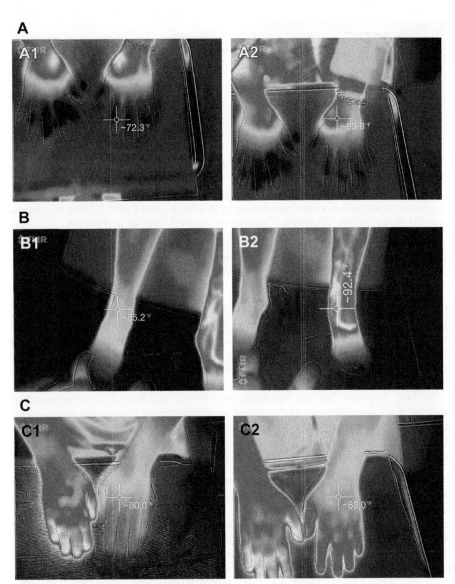

Fig. 2. (*A*) Secondary Raynaud syndrome and Lupus with 11.5°F difference between proximal hand (*A1*) (*left image*) and distal digits (*A2*) (*right image*). (*B*) Pseudogout attack in left ankle (*left image*) (*B1*), 7.2°F difference with right ankle (*B2*). (*C*) Takayasu arteritis and left subclavian artery stenosis with sedimentation rate of 113 mm/h (*left image*) (*C1*), after 2 months of high-dose corticosteroids, 7.2°F difference with sedimentation rate, reduced to 13 mm/h (*right image*) (*C2*).

to 3 weeks, requiring users to engage 10 to 15 minutes per day for audio-based sessions.

Technology adoption for the office-based physician is (and continues) to be driven by the smartphone. The ideal office technology needs to be affordable, usable, fast, and aid patient outcomes. More research is needed to see if additional technology products can significantly affect diagnosis and management. Along with hardware, software can be used for productivity, education, informed consent, and to manage comorbidities. Increasingly, patients are using data and technology to help manage their illness but welcome physician guidance.

SUMMARY

Although the advent of digital medicine has been slow to take hold, the pace of adaptation of digital medicine will accelerate over the next several years. Advances in biosensors, artificial intelligence, telemedicine, VR, smart monitors etc. are going to transform the way that medicine will be practiced. Digital medicine provides rheumatology many opportunities to innovate and redefine the way we practice medicine. In addition, tools that help us achieve these goals will become more pervasive. Although change is inevitable, it will require us as rheumatologists to define the basic questions of who these interventions will be helpful for, when they are worth using, where interventions should be administered, and perhaps most importantly, will these new technologies help provide better, safer, and cheaper care for our patients.

ACKNOWLEDGEMENTS

We would like to acknowledge Timothy Chu, BS for writing assistance, final proofreading, and organization of cited sources which contributed to the overall quality of the final paper.

REFERENCES

1. Health IT. Office-based physician electronic health record adoption. 2015. Available at: https://dashboard.healthit.gov/quickstats/pages/physician-ehr-adoption-trends.php. Accessed July 16, 2018.
2. Steinhubl SR, Topol EJ. Digital medicine, on its way to being just plain medicine. NPJ Digit Med 2018;1(1):20175.
3. Pew Research Center. Demographics of mobile device ownership and adoption in the United States. 2018. Available at: http://www.pewinternet.org/fact-sheet/mobile/. Accessed July 11, 2018.
4. Pew Research Center. Demographics of social media users and adoption in the United States. 2018. Available at: http://www.pewinternet.org/fact-sheet/social-media/. Accessed July 11, 2018.
5. Campion EW, Scott L, Graham A, et al. NEJM.org - 20 years on the web. N Engl J Med 2016;375(10):993–4.
6. Ibrahim AM. Seeing is believing: using visual abstracts to disseminate scientific research. Am J Gastroenterol 2018;113(4):459–61.
7. Hausmann JS, Doss J, Cappelli L. Use of social media by rheumatology fellows in North America: abstract Number: 1012. Arthritis Rheumatol 2015;67:1321–3.
8. Nikiphorou E, Studenic P, Ammitzboll CG, et al. Social media use among young rheumatologists and basic scientists: results of an international survey by the Emerging EULAR Network (EMEUNET). Ann Rheum Dis 2017;76(4):712–5.
9. Collins C, Campos J, Isabelle A, et al. AB1385 #rheumjc: 3 year analysis of a twitter based rheumatology journal club. Annals of the Rheumatic Diseases 2018;77:1777.
10. Mohameden M, Malkhasyan V, Alkhairi B, et al. Tweeting the meeting: analysis of twitter use during the American College of Rheumatology 2016 annual meeting. Paper presented at: Arthritis & Rheumatology. November 11-16, 2016

11. Colbert GB, Topf J, Jhaveri KD, et al. The social media revolution in nephrology education. Kidney Int Rep 2018;3(3):519–29.
12. Berenbaum F. The social (media) side to rheumatology. Nat Rev Rheumatol 2014; 10(5):314–8.
13. Twitter. Rheumatology A public list by American College of Rheumatology. 2018. Available at: https://twitter.com/acrheum?lang=en. Accessed July 11, 2018.
14. Symplur. The healthcare hashtag project. 2018. Available at: https://www.symplur.com/healthcare-hashtags/. Accessed July 11, 2018.
15. Amigues I, Sufka P, Bhana S, et al. # Rheumjc: impact of invited authors on a twitter based rheumatology journal club. Paper presented at: Arthritis & Rheumatology. November 11-16, 2016.
16. Kalia V, Ortiz DA, Patel AK, et al. Leveraging twitter to maximize the radiology meeting experience. J Am Coll Radiol 2018;15(1):177–83.
17. Logghe HJ, Selby LV, Boeck MA, et al. The academic tweet: Twitter as a tool to advance academic surgery. J Surg Res 2018;226. viii–xii.
18. Cawcutt K. Twitter me this—can social media revolutionize academic medicine? Infect Control Hosp Epidemiol 2017;38(12):1501–2.
19. Cabrera D, Vartabedian BS, Spinner RJ, et al. More than likes and tweets: creating social media portfolios for academic promotion and tenure. J Grad Med Educ 2017;9(4):421–5.
20. Altmetric. Discover the attention surrounding your research. 2018. Available at: https://www.altmetric.com/. Accessed July 11, 2018.
21. Altmetric. What are altmetrics? 2018. Available at: https://www.altmetric.com/about-altmetrics/what-are-altmetrics/. Accessed July 11, 2018.
22. Trueger NS, Thoma B, Hsu CH, et al. The altmetric score: a new measure for article-level dissemination and impact. Ann Emerg Med 2015;66(5):549–53.
23. Wiley. Promotional toolkit for authors. 2018. Available at: https://authorservices.wiley.com/author-resources/Journal-Authors/Promotion/promotional-toolkit.html. Accessed July 11, 2018.
24. Wright P. 5 tips for improving your article's Altmetric score, Vol 2018. The Wiley Network; 2014. Available at: https://hub.wiley.com/community/exchanges/discover/blog/2014/09/18/5-tips-for-improving-your-articles-altmetric-score.
25. Mendeley. Empowering researchers to store and share their data. 2018. Available at: https://www.mendeley.com/. Accessed July 11, 2018.
26. Chan TM, Stukus D, Leppink J, et al. Social media and the 21st-century scholar: how you can harness social media to amplify your career. J Am Coll Radiol 2018; 15(1 Pt B):142–8.
27. Shillcutt SK, Silver JK. Social media and advancement of women physicians. N Engl J Med 2018;378(24):2342–5.
28. Kind T. Professional guidelines for social media use: a starting point. AMA J Ethics 2015;17(5):441–7.
29. Mayo Clinic. Social for healthcare certificate from mayo clinic and hootsuite. 2018. Available at: https://socialmedia.mayoclinic.org/social-media-basics-certification/#. Accessed July 11, 2018.
30. Rosen A. Tweeting made easier. vol. 2018. 2017. Available at: blog.twitter.
31. Twitter. How to create a thread on twitter. 2018. Available at: https://help.twitter.com/en/using-twitter/create-a-thread. Accessed July 11, 2018.
32. Vartabedian BS. Long-form twitter and the physician conversation 2018. Available at: https://33charts.com/long-form-twitter-physician/. Accessed July 11, 2018.

33. Gerardi M, Cukor J, Difede J, et al. Virtual reality exposure therapy for post-traumatic stress disorder and other anxiety disorders. Curr Psychiatry Rep 2010;12(4):298–305.
34. Rudd RA, Seth P, David F, et al. Increases in drug and opioid-involved overdose deaths - United States, 2010-2015. MMWR Morb Mortal Wkly Rep 2016;65(5051):1445–52.
35. Mahan KT. The opioid crisis. J Foot Ankle Surg 2017;56(1):1–2.
36. McCaul KD, Malott JM. Distraction and coping with pain. Psychol Bull 1984;95(3):516–33.
37. Hoffman HG, Patterson DR, Carrougher GJ, et al. Effectiveness of virtual reality-based pain control with multiple treatments. Clin J Pain 2001;17(3):229–35.
38. Botella C, Garcia-Palacios A, Vizcaino Y, et al. Virtual reality in the treatment of fibromyalgia: a pilot study. Cyberpsychol Behav Soc Netw 2013;16(3):215–23.
39. Li A, Montano Z, Chen VJ, et al. Virtual reality and pain management: current trends and future directions. Pain Manag 2011;1(2):147–57.
40. Gold JI, Belmont KA, Thomas DA. The neurobiology of virtual reality pain attenuation. Cyberpsychol Behav 2007;10(4):536–44.
41. Hoffman HG, Richards TL, Van Oostrom T, et al. The analgesic effects of opioids and immersive virtual reality distraction: evidence from subjective and functional brain imaging assessments. Anesth Analg 2007;105(6):1776–83. Table of contents.
42. Hoffman HG, Patterson DR, Seibel E, et al. Virtual reality pain control during burn wound debridement in the hydrotank. Clin J Pain 2008;24(4):299–304.
43. Pourmand A, Davis S, Marchak A, et al. Virtual reality as a clinical tool for pain management. Curr Pain Headache Rep 2018;22(8):53.
44. Thomas JS, France CR, Applegate ME, et al. Feasibility and safety of a virtual reality dodgeball intervention for chronic low back pain: a randomized clinical trial. J Pain 2016;17(12):1302–17.
45. Morris LD, Louw QA, Grimmer KA, et al. Targeting pain catastrophization in patients with fibromyalgia using virtual reality exposure therapy: a proof-of-concept study. J Phys Ther Sci 2015;27(11):3461–7.
46. Garcia-Palacios A, Herrero R, Vizcaino Y, et al. Integrating virtual reality with activity management for the treatment of fibromyalgia: acceptability and preliminary efficacy. Clin J Pain 2015;31(6):564–72.
47. Gokeler A, Bisschop M, Myer GD, et al. Immersive virtual reality improves movement patterns in patients after ACL reconstruction: implications for enhanced criteria-based return-to-sport rehabilitation. Knee Surg Sports Traumatol Arthrosc 2016;24(7):2280–6.
48. Kim J, Son J, Ko N, et al. Unsupervised virtual reality-based exercise program improves hip muscle strength and balance control in older adults: a pilot study. Arch Phys Med Rehabil 2013;94(5):937–43.
49. Wagner K. Facebook-owned oculus built another VR headset: the $199 wireless 'Oculus Go'. 2017. Available at: https://www.recode.net/2017/10/11/16459432/facebook-mark-zuckerberg-oculus-go-virtual-reality-headset-launch-rift-cost. Accessed July 16, 2018.
50. Medicine V. Virtual medicine: best practices in medical virtual reality. 2018. Available at: https://www.virtualmedicine.health/. Accessed August 6, 2018.
51. Twitter. Brennan Spiegel, MD. 2018. Available at: https://twitter.com/BrennanSpiegel?ref_src=twsrc%5Egoogle%7Ctwcamp%5Eserp%7Ctwgr%5Eauthor. Accessed August 6, 2018.

52. The Medical Futurist. Virtual reality is used in clinical practice. 2017. Available at: https://medicalfuturist.com/virtual-reality-used-clinical-practice/. Accessed July 16, 2018.

53. Hama M, Takase K, Ihata A, et al. Challenges to expanding the clinical application of musculoskeletal ultrasonography (MSUS) among rheumatologists: from a second survey in Japan. Mod Rheumatol 2012;22(2):202–8.

54. Larche MJ, McDonald-Blumer H, Bruns A, et al. Utility and feasibility of musculoskeletal ultrasonography (MSK US) in rheumatology practice in Canada: needs assessment. Clin Rheumatol 2011;30(10):1277–83.

55. Speier W, Dzubur E, Zide M, et al. Evaluating utility and compliance in a patient-based eHealth study using continuous-time heart rate and activity trackers. J Am Med Inform Assoc 2018;25(10):1386–91.

56. Colver K. A11 bionic chip in iPhone 8 and iPhone X on par with 13-Inch MacBook Pro, outperforms iPad Pro. 2017. Available at: https://www.macrumors.com/2017/09/13/a11-bionic-chip-geekbench-scores/. Accessed July 11, 2018.

57. Cutolo M, Pizzorni C, Secchi ME, et al. Capillaroscopy. Best Pract Res Clin Rheumatol 2008;22(6):1093–108.

58. Sanchez BM, Lesch M, Brammer D, et al. Use of a portable thermal imaging unit as a rapid, quantitative method of evaluating inflammation and experimental arthritis. J Pharmacol Toxicol Methods 2008;57(3):169–75.

59. Frize M, Ogungbemile A. Estimating rheumatoid arthritis activity with infrared image analysis. Stud Health Technol Inform 2012;180:594–8.

60. Neogi T, Jansen TL, Dalbeth N, et al. 2015 Gout classification criteria: an American College of Rheumatology/European League Against Rheumatism collaborative initiative. Ann Rheum Dis 2015;74(10):1789–98.

61. Markman TM, Sampognaro PJ, Mitchell SL, et al. Medical student appraisal: applications for bedside patient education. Appl Clin Inform 2013;4(2):201–11.

62. Athilingam P, Osorio RE, Kaplan H, et al. Embedding patient education in mobile platform for patients with heart failure: theory-based development and beta testing. Comput Inform Nurs 2016;34(2):92–8.

63. Health NIo. Pain management. 2010. Available at: https://report.nih.gov/nihfactsheets/ViewFactSheet.aspx?csid=57. Accessed July 16, 2018.

64. Sharon H, Maron-Katz A, Ben Simon E, et al. Mindfulness meditation modulates pain through endogenous opioids. Am J Med 2016;129(7):755–8.

65. Zeidan F, Emerson NM, Farris SR, et al. Mindfulness meditation-based pain relief employs different neural mechanisms than placebo and sham mindfulness meditation-induced analgesia. J Neurosci 2015;35(46):15307–25.

Challenges in Optimizing Medical Education for Rheumatologists

Sian Yik Lim, MD[a,*], Marcy B. Bolster, MD[b]

KEYWORDS

- Medical education • Continuing medical education • Rheumatology fellowship

KEY POINTS

- The field of rheumatology has expanded rapidly in recent years, and innovations in immunology, epigenetics, and bone metabolism continue at an astonishing pace.
- In the fast-changing rheumatology field, optimizing medical education for rheumatologists is vital for maintaining a competent workforce to meet the needs of patients with rheumatic diseases.
- A multifaceted approach is warranted to optimize medical education for rheumatologists across the career span.
- Medical education for rheumatologists in the future has to involve all stages in the development of a well-trained rheumatologist, readying the fellow for practice, effectively transitioning from fellowship to practice, and promoting lifelong learning in rheumatology.

INTRODUCTION

The field of rheumatology has expanded rapidly in recent years, and innovations in immunology, epigenetics, and bone metabolism continue at an astonishing pace. In this fast-changing field, optimizing medical education for rheumatologists is vital for maintaining a competent workforce to meet the needs of patients with rheumatic diseases. Several key challenges lie ahead. For example, the 2015 American College of Rheumatology (ACR) Workforce Study projected a shortage of adult rheumatologists accompanied by a significant increase in patient demand over the next decade.[1] Although narrowing the gap between supply of and demand for rheumatology care, optimization of cost-effective care and ongoing quality improvement efforts remain fundamental.[2] Rapid developments in the etiopathogenesis of rheumatic disease, awareness of the role of comorbidities, evolving knowledge of prognostic factors

[a] Bone and Joint Department, Straub Clinic, 800 South King Street, Honolulu, HI 96813, USA;
[b] Division of Rheumatology, Allergy, and Immunology, Harvard Medical School, Rheumatology Fellowship Training Program, Massachusetts General Hospital, 55 Fruit Street, Boston, MA 02114, USA
* Corresponding author.
E-mail address: limsianyik@gmail.com

Rheum Dis Clin N Am 45 (2019) 127–144
https://doi.org/10.1016/j.rdc.2018.09.008
0889-857X/19/© 2018 Elsevier Inc. All rights reserved.
rheumatic.theclinics.com

affecting clinical outcomes, and the increasing availability of new treatments have made lifelong learning a critical part of rheumatology practice.[3] The change in work-force demographics,[4] the rapid growth of medical discovery, new expectations for patient care, and ongoing efforts to improve quality of care pose meaningful challenges that need to be addressed by efforts to optimize medical education.

ADULT LEARNING THEORY

Adult learning theory provides guidance on meeting the challenges of educating rheumatologists. No single theory is explanatory, but several principles form an important framework to guide both fellowship education and the lifelong learning important to rheumatology practice.[5]

The concept andragogy, described by Knowles, highlights the differences in learning between adults and children. Andradogy is based on the premise that attainment of adulthood is represented by individuals viewing themselves as self-directed. The characteristics of adult learning include self-direction, autonomy in learning, problem-centered learning, and learning based on the accumulated reservoir of life experiences, goals, and objectives.[6] Other adult learning theories that describe learning characteristics include Jarvis's learning process, which highlights life experience as a significant quality in adult learning. Reflective learning is an important concept, as it allows physicians to test and review underlying beliefs through a process of reflection and action. Transformative learning theory describes a learning method in which critical reflection is used to challenge the learner's beliefs and assumptions, leading to internalizing a revised interpretation of the meaning of one's experience as guide to future actions.[7]

Fundamental to these theories and concepts, the education of rheumatologists should be based on the premise that the learner is an active contributor in the process, importantly, including reflection and self-regulation (the ability to understand and control one's learning environment). Clear learning objectives, a focus on tasks that can be performed, and problem solving pertinent to clinical practice provide a strong educational foundation.[5] It is also important to take into account the learners' knowledge and past experiences, as well as their values, attitudes, and beliefs toward learning.[7]

OPTIMIZING EDUCATION FOR THE RHEUMATOLOGIST

The following sections describe critical stages of optimizing medical education, including fellow readiness for practice, transitioning from training to practice, and lifelong learning. **Table 1**, while not all-inclusive, describes many important resources that can be utilized in these processes.

Readying the Fellow for Practice

Standardized core curriculum

One of the critical challenges of optimizing medical education for the rheumatologist is the readying of the fellow for practice. The foundation of this preparation is fellowship training. It is crucial to provide high-quality standardized training during fellowship to serve as the groundwork for future multifaceted career development.

Fellowship training In the United States, formal rheumatology fellowship training consists of a 2-year training program accredited by the American College of Graduate Medical Education (ACGME). Upon completion of fellowship training, graduates are

Table 1 Resources for optimizing rheumatology education	
Resource	**Description**
The Rheumatology Core Curriculum Outline	• Detailed guide for rheumatology program directors to utilize in the development of a fellowship training curriculum • Based on ACGME core competencies focusing on competency-based training and assessment in graduate medical education
Rheumatology In-training Examination	• Standardized Web-based examination administered by fellowship programs to enable each fellow to assess medical knowledge and compare results against national outcomes; it also provides program directors with information on strengths and gaps in the fellowship program curriculum
Ultrasound School of North American Rheumatologists (USSONAR)	• An 8-month program that combines internet-based instruction, a hands-on workshop, and testing of ultrasound learning designed to provide musculoskeletal ultrasound training
The Rheumatology Musculoskeletal Ultrasound Certification Pathway (RhMSUS)	• Independent verification of musculoskeletal expertise for rheumatologists by the American College of Rheumatology
Quality Bone Densitometry: Performance, Interpretation, and Clinical Application for Clinicians	• A 2-day course providing instruction for interpretation of bone densitometry in children and adults
Clinical Certified Densitometrist	• Independent verification of knowledge of interpretation of bone mineral density by the International Society of Clinical Densitometry
American College of Rheumatology Annual Meeting	• Largest annual meeting of the American College of Rheumatology with opportunities for professional development, presentations of the latest research, and networking
American College of Rheumatology State-of the Art Clinical Symposium (SOTA)	• Annual meeting offering information about clinical best practices and evidence-based treatment in rheumatology.
Coalition of State Rheumatology Organizations Fellows Conference	• Conference for rheumatology fellows providing information about career development and skills essential to community practice (contract negotiation, coding, and practice management)
Body of Knowledge for Medical Practice Management	• A resource published by the Medical Group Management Association that defines all important areas of knowledge and skills needed to run a successful medical practice

(*continued on next page*)

Table 1 (continued)	
Resource	Description
American College of Rheumatology Continuing Assessment Review Evaluation (CARE)	• Modules consisting of multiple choice questions covering rheumatology topics within the American Board of Internal Medicine blueprint
American College of Rheumatology Image Bank	• A collection of images over a wide range of rheumatic diseases

eligible for rheumatology board certification, a secure examination of multiple choice questions administered by the American Board of Internal Medicine.

The ACR Core Curriculum mission statement outlines that "the goal of fellowship training is to train fellows that: (1) are clinically competent in the field of rheumatology, (2) are capable of working in a variety of settings, and (3) possess habits of lifelong learning to build upon their knowledge, skills, and professionalism."[8] Based on this charge, each rheumatology fellowship program develops its goals and objectives of training. In most rheumatology fellowship training programs, the first year is designed to provide in-depth clinical training across a broad spectrum of clinical rheumatology.[9,10] The second year of fellowship training builds upon the foundation developed in the first year to sharpen the fellow's clinical skills. Furthermore, during the second year, many fellowship programs provide reduced clinical exposure for fellows in order to introduce rigorous scientific training. Fellows planning to pursue an academic career may pursue additional years of training, beyond the ACGME-required 2 years of training, in order to delve deeper into clinical or basic science research.

Resources for fellowship education Outlined below are some of the important resources used for fellow education in the United States.

Rheumatology Core Curriculum The ACR has an updated core curriculum outline for fellowship training that provides a homogeneous foundation for fellow education. Endorsed by the ACR, this outline provides a detailed guide for rheumatology fellowship program directors to utilize in the development of each institution's fellowship training curriculum.[9] The core curriculum outline was updated In June 2015, based on the 2006 ACR Core Curriculum Outline for Program Directors (2006). It is organized using the ACGME core competencies (**Box 1**). The core curriculum highlights the importance of competency-based training and assessment in graduate medical education, and this represents a shift from the traditional model of medical education.

Box 1 American College of Graduate Medical Education core competencies
• Medical Knowledge
• Patient care and procedural skills
• Systems-based practice
• Practice-based learning and improvement
• Interpersonal and communication skills
• Professionalism

Competency-based training and assessment are discussed in more detail in subsequent sections.

Rheum4Science The ACR has recently introduced an online resource comprised of interactive modules to enhance basic science and clinical research exposure and education for rheumatology fellows.[11] Although Rheum4Science is being developed for use in fellowship education, its applicability and appeal are more far-reaching and can be utilized by any rheumatology learner.

Rheumatology In-Training Examination The Rheumatology In-Training Examination (ITE) is a standardized, secure, Web-based examination consisting of 200 multiple choice questions, developed each year by the ACR In-Training Examination Subcommittee of the ACR Committee on Training and Workforce (COTW), with the support of the National Board of Medical Examiners.[12] The ITE enables each fellow to assess his or her medical knowledge and compare his or her results against national outcomes reported, by year in training, in the score reports.[13] The ITE allows each program director to identify areas of strength and weakness in his or her training program curriculum. Thus, based on fellow performance on the ITE, in addition to a fellow creating a targeted reading program for areas of weakness, a program director can bolster certain areas of the training curriculum to strengthen fellow education. This can be accomplished through conference topics, focused discussions at point of patient care, and special sessions to address knowledge gaps.

American Board of Internal Medicine board preparation and certification American Board of Internal Medicine (ABIM) Rheumatology board certification is designed to evaluate knowledge, diagnostic reasoning, and clinical judgment skills expected of a board-certified rheumatologist.[14] Examination content is based on an established and updated blueprint that is reviewed annually by the ABIM Rheumatology Exam Committee.[14] Fellows who have completed 2 years of ACGME-accredited fellowship training are eligible to take the examination, and upon passing, become ABIM Rheumatology board certified.

Board preparation and certification require a multifaceted approach, built upon the trainee's didactic, clinical learning experience, and broad reading of rheumatology textbooks and primary literature during fellowship training. Board preparation materials can help solidify knowledge acquired and orient the trainee toward the board examination format. Board preparation materials may be sought depending on the trainee's learning style.

Created by an ACR subcommittee, the Continuing Assessment Review Evaluation (CARE) modules are an important resource for board certification preparation. These modules consist of multiple choice questions covering rheumatology topics within the ABIM blueprint. The ACR Image Bank provides a collection of images over a range of rheumatic diseases, which can be helpful in board preparation. Rheumatology ITE performance predicts performance on the ABIM Rheumatology Board Certification examination. Therefore, the adult rheumatology ITE can be used to provide feedback to direct the fellow's learning toward board certification.[13] There are other board preparation courses and materials available for attendance and purchase, respectively, as offered by academic institutions across the United States.

Tailoring Education Based on the Fellow's Interests and Needs

Based on a solid foundation from the Rheumatology Core Curriculum Outline, optimizing education for rheumatologists must account for personal interests and individual career goals. Professional goals differ for rheumatology fellows transitioning to academic clinical faculty compared with those entering community practice. Therefore, a tailored, individualized educational approach, built on the foundation of the core curriculum, is important in order to best meet these needs. Although fellows entering academic clinical practice and community practice may have many shared educational goals and aspirations for creating a niche in clinical practice, there are some areas of identified need in promoting a fellow to most effectively and efficiently integrate into community practice.

Musculoskeletal ultrasound training

Musculoskeletal ultrasound (MSUS) is increasingly used in the care of patients with rheumatic diseases and musculoskeletal disorders. Most rheumatology fellowship training programs incorporate some format of MSUS training in their curriculum, although there remains significant variability among programs regarding the depth of MSUS education provided.[15] Efforts are ongoing to develop a formal curriculum for MSUS training in fellowship. In a study published in 2017, the percentage of programs teaching MSUS and the percentage of those with a formal curriculum were 94% and 41%, respectively.[15] Notably, MSUS teaching has increased from 41% in a 2008 survey; however, programs implementing a formal curriculum have been unchanged over this time period.[16]

External courses, such as the Ultrasound School of North American Rheumatologists (USSONAR) program, have been utilized by many fellowship programs to supplement their own MSUS training. The USSONAR program combines Internet-based instruction (short online teaching modules and mentor-provided feedback on submitted scans), a hands-on workshop (hands-on cadaver-based injection training), and testing of ultrasound learning (written examination and objective structured scanning examination) to optimize MSUS education among rheumatologists.[15,17] Postfellowship rheumatologists also have the opportunity to participate in the USSONAR program.

The Rheumatology Musculoskeletal Ultrasound (RhMSUS) Certification pathway, offered by the American College of Rheumatology, provides independent verification of musculoskeletal expertise for rheumatologists.[15] RhMSUS certification requires submission of 150 ultrasound scans, completion of continuing medical education (CME) activities in MSUS, and passing a written examination.[15,18] The USSONAR program is a separate entity from the RhMSUS, and USSONAR does not provide certification.[18] However, completion of the USSONAR program is one of the pathways that can be taken for RhMSUS certification.

Dual-energy x-ray absorptiometry interpretation

Rheumatology fellowship programs teach dual-energy x-ray absorptiometry (DXA) interpretation to varying degrees as part of a broader bone health curriculum. The International Society of Clinical Densitometry (ISCD) conducts courses, accredited for certified clinical densitometists (CCDs), covering uses and interpretation of DXA scans in the management of a patient's bone health.[19] For fellows transitioning to clinical practice, either in academics or community practice, determination should be individualized for the need for more advanced DXA interpretation skills, and thus for certification, in providing outpatient care for patients with rheumatic disease. Similarly, once in practice, rheumatologists can choose to pursue DXA interpretation certification through ISCD training.

Infusion center practice

Rheumatologists prescribe infusible disease-modifying agents for a broad spectrum of conditions including autoimmune, inflammatory, metabolic, and osteoporosis in the treatment of patients with rheumatic diseases. Because of the increasing number of infusible medications, infusion center patient care and practice management have become an essential aspect of clinical rheumatology practice. Many rheumatologists are called upon to manage acute infusion reactions, but unfortunately many fellowship programs do not have a formal curriculum to address this important area.[20] Weiner and colleagues[20] implemented an innovative brief, intensive curriculum involving objective structured clinical examination (OSCE) of a simulated experience of an on-call rheumatologist paged by an infusion center nurse about a patient having an acute infusion reaction. The OSCE was followed by 3 minutes of face-to-face feedback and included a separate 15-minute didactic session with pre- and post-tests assessing attitudes, comfort, and knowledge about infusion reactions. This teaching session was well-received and found to be effective in educating rheumatologists on the management of acute infusion reactions.[20] Although infusion center practice has become an critical part of rheumatology practice, literature regarding infusion practices by rheumatologists is scarce. Management of an infusion center practice requires practice management skills, as described in the following section, as well as mastery of specific knowledge regarding billing, coding and compliance for infusions services, medications infused, and managing the logistics of the infusion services provided.[21,22]

Practice management

Medical education literature regarding practice management in rheumatology is limited. However, several efforts in other specialties have resulted in publication of approaches to education in medical practice. Wichman and colleagues[23] developed a 32-week didactic curriculum in a psychiatry residency program based on domains described by the American College of Medical Practice Executives (ACMPE) and the Medical Group Management Association (MGMA). Other programs combine didactics exposing physicians to the business aspect of medicine with hands-on experience with administrative rotations.[24] Other approaches include involving full-time business educators within the training program,[25] and weekend retreats focusing on business aspects of medicine.[26] In terms of rheumatology preparedness for practice, the ACR offers sessions on practice management at its annual meeting and during the fellows' sessions at the ACR State of the Art Meeting (SOTA). Although there may be other opportunities on a local or state level, the Coalition of State Rheumatology Organizations conducts an annual conference providing information to fellows who will transition to clinical practice. The conference focuses on career development and skills essential to community practice, including contract negotiation, coding, and other matters that may not be covered in depth during fellowship training. Continued efforts are needed in rheumatology training programs to enhance fellows' exposure to the business aspect of rheumatology practice to best prepare for the transition to practice.

Transitions: Launch from Fellowship

The transition from fellowship to practice, whether to community practice or to an academic position, is an important step for each rheumatologist. Successfully navigating this transition is one of the challenges in medical education for rheumatologists. Notably, there are many different career tracks available; however, in general, the most significant branch point in decision-making is whether to pursue community practice or academic medicine.

Transition to Community Practice

Transitioning to community practice presents several unique challenges for the fellow. One of the difficulties many fellows face is the knowledge gap for the business of medicine and contractual aspects of securing a job. Although the ACGME acknowledges the importance of practice management, through the systems-based practice competency, practice management is absent or not a significant part of the curriculum for many rheumatology fellowship training programs.[23] For physicians transitioning to community practice, business management and infusion practice management, as previously described, are vital.

The ACR provides valuable practice management resources, including updated information on practice management, clinical practice guidelines, insurance advocacy, and regulations. The ACR has several publications and resources for practice management, including "The Business Side of Rheumatology Practice" and a "Rheumatology Coding Manual," providing useful references to learn about practice management.[27] The ACR Practice Management Team also organizes courses such as the Advanced Rheumatology Coding & Clinical Documentation Improvement Boot Camp and the Certified Rheumatology Coder Review Course & Exam to help provide rheumatologists with updated information about practice management.[28]

The MGMA publishes the "Body of Knowledge (BOK) for Medical Practice Management," which serves as an important guide and useful learning tool for medical practice management.[29] As a fundamental resource, it defines all important areas of knowledge and skills needed to run a successful medical practice. The 4 necessary competencies to excel at practice management include professionalism, leadership, communications skills, and organizational and analytical skills. The domains covered in the current body of knowledge include financial management, human resources management, organizational governance, operations management, patient-centered care, and risk and compliance management.[29]

In addition to practice management resources, the rheumatologist has several options for learning about the business of practice management during the transition period to community practice. Master's degree programs include master of business administration or other master's degrees such as masters of health administration and masters of medical management.[30] Certificate programs and shorter introductory courses are offered by the American College of Health Care Executives and American College of Medical Practice Executives (ACPME) to better enable physicians to learn about the business aspect of rheumatology.[30]

One of the key endeavors in clinical practice is the systematic, formal approach to the analysis of practice performance and efforts to improve performance–quality improvement.[31] Essential steps in a quality improvement project include determination of potential areas for improvement, collection and analysis of data, reporting results, and commitment to ongoing evaluation. The processes employed include Model for Improvement (Plan-Do-Study-Act cycles), Six Sigma, and Lean. Implementation of quality improvement contributes to a well-functioning practice, and its implementation also helps improve clinic productivity, patient safety, and clinical outcomes. Quality improvement projects, an ACGME requirement in training, are also essential for practicing clinicians to participate in federal quality payment programs.[31] Although many training programs lack formal training, a structured quality improvement curriculum, in collaboration with faculty who are proficient in quality improvement, is a key way to optimize rheumatology education in preparation for the transition to practice.[32]

Transition to Academic Clinical Faculty

Although the clinical and research mentorship in fellowship training is not only acknowledged, but is generally robust, one of the challenges in the transition from fellow to academic rheumatology is the lack of mentorship for career development. In a study of 162 junior faculty consisting of those in the clinician-scientist and clinician-educator tracks, less than 50% of new faculty reported feeling adequately mentored.[33] Successful mentoring programs lead to increased levels of teaching effectiveness, research productivity, and satisfaction with one's career.[34]

Mentorship in the transition from fellow to faculty likely occurs to a greater extent in the scientific investigation arenas, either clinical or bench science research, than for those rheumatologists with a greater focus on clinical practice in the academic setting. Professional development for clinicians in academic practice is also of importance in terms of developing clinical expertise, speaking and teaching opportunities, leadership positions, involvement with national societies, and academic promotion. Evidence supports the benefits of establishing formal mentoring programs, compared with informal systems.[34] Therefore, it is critical that academic programs continue to develop and refine formal mentoring systems in an effort to enhance education in rheumatology as well as to retain rheumatologists in academic positions.

A formal mentoring system may be implemented by the Rheumatology Division, the Department of Medicine, or at the institutional level. It can be comprised by many facets of mentorship, including but not limited to mentor-mentee assignments for one-on-one guidance, grant writing assistance, networking within the institution, as well as regionally and nationally, committee participation, requiring junior faculty to report to mentoring committees to help define individualized goals and timelines, and facilitation of participation of young investigators in team science meetings, conference calls, and disease-focused multicenter interest groups.[35]

Utilization of external resources including resources from the ACR and the parent academic institution may be helpful, especially for smaller rheumatology programs that may not be able to sustain a formal mentorship program. For example, the ACR and the Childhood Arthritis and Rheumatology Research Alliance (CARRA) developed the ACR/CARRA Mentoring Interest Group (AMIGO) to facilitate mentoring of junior pediatric rheumatology faculty. AMIGO organizes educational and networking sessions to promote a culture of mentorship. Furthermore, an innovative mentoring program was developed to match mentees with mentors from other institutions.[36] When surveyed, participants in the mentorship program noted benefits in career development, scholarship, job satisfaction, and an increased connection to the academic community.[36] Mentors also reported gains in their mentoring skills and academic portfolios.[36]

Another challenge of the transition to academic faculty is facilitating a focus on the traditional core missions of academic health centers, research, education, and clinical care.[37] Because of the rapid advancement of medical science and increased complexity of clinical care, academic institutions have moved away from the traditional model in which the faculty member was expected to be a triple threat and excel in all roles of being a clinician, educator, and scientific investigator.[37] Clinicians at academic centers pursue the clinician educator or the clinician scientist pathway; physicians in both pathways are involved in clinical care, to a varying extent.

The ability to focus on medical education, clinical, or basic science research requires funding to ensure protected time for young faculty to develop skills in teaching and research. Funding attainment remains a significant barrier to the successful transition from trainee to academic faculty. For rheumatologists on the clinical investigator track, new investigators seek support from "K" awards from the National Institutes of Health (NIH). These are 5-year grants providing a research salary, and this award helps to foster mentored career development as a research investigator. In recent years, because of decreased NIH funding, the granting of "K" awards has decreased by 23% to 48%.[35] Notably, NIH funding for established investigators has declined also, including a 30% decrease in the number of individual investigator RO1 grants for ACR members.[35] Concerted efforts are needed to increase and diversify sources of funding to support rheumatology research. Foundation funding, especially from the Rheumatology Research Foundation, has become a significant source of funding for young rheumatologists pursuing a research career.[35] Other vital sources of funding include disease-related foundations, pharmaceutical companies, and philanthropic sources.

Lifelong Learning in Rheumatology

Although formal training concludes with the end of fellowship, clearly ongoing rheumatology education persists throughout the career lifetime. Learning in medicine is a lifelong process, and while learning during fellowship years is termed training, the wealth gained from continuing medical education (CME), both informal and formal, is enriching and rewarding and is an essential component of physician education and practice.

Multiple Demands on the Practicing Rheumatologist

Promoting lifelong learning in rheumatology must take into account the numerous demands and challenges of the busy practicing rheumatologist. One of the most significant constraints for the busy clinician is incorporating CME activities into a busy clinical schedule. Besides the daily duties of clinical work, many clinicians need to balance their time with administrative tasks and family responsibilities and activities, often leading to loss of interest or insufficient time to commit to participating in CME activities.[38] Many rheumatology practices are small in size; therefore, they may not have the ability to support structured CME activities specific to rheumatology.[38] Traveling to CME conferences involves significant expense, including travel and registration costs. Furthermore, CME meeting attendance results in a reduction in productivity revenue while overhead continues in the clinician's absence.

Resources for Lifelong Learning

Textbooks and journal articles

Traditional resources for the most current medical knowledge include rheumatology textbooks and journal articles, now enjoying greater online accessibility. Journal articles are easily accessible and searchable at the point of care through PubMed, a free full-text archive of biomedical and life sciences journal literature at the NIH's National Library of Medicine.[39] Online clinical knowledge support systems such as UpToDate, DynaMed, and Clinical Key are increasingly popular for physicians to aid in staying current with medical knowledge and can easily be utilized at the point of care, thus immediately available at the time and location where needed.[40,41] The immediacy of information availability enables the clinician to deepen his or her knowledge about a specific clinical condition or patient-related question and allows the rheumatologist to provide enhanced medical care. Although online resources provide immediate access, with the patient in the examination room, often more in-depth reading is warranted regarding the patient's condition. Depending on the complexity of the question being explored, a textbook or the primary literature provides a sound basis for clinician learning and for optimizing patient care. By utilizing textbooks and/or the primary literature to address a patient care dilemma, these resources augment clinician learning, because adult learning occurs most efficiently when the educational process is coupled with a relevant specific activity or clinical problem.

Social media platforms

Social media are comprised of computer-mediated technologies, facilitating the creation and sharing of information and ideas via virtual communities and social networking services.[42] Popular social networking services include Twitter, Facebook, and YouTube, all of which allow the inexpensive and efficient sharing of information while producing value.[43] An increasing body of evidence shows that social media platforms provide an effective strategy for dissemination of clinical evidence, research findings, and drug safety communications to providers.[44–48] Social media tools allow health care professionals to receive the latest information pertaining to their professional interests. This is easily accomplished by subscribing to and following updates from social network accounts of major journals or professional associations.

Social media can also be utilized as a powerful tool to actively engage a learner and provide real-time education. For example, in a prospective cohort study, pharmacists tweeted infectious disease topics relevant to surgeons in an effort to provide education about antimicrobial stewardship. Almost 77% of the surgeons found that the information presented was relevant to their practice.[49] Social media, by facilitating communication, strengthens professional interactions and relationships. For example, Twitter-based journal clubs provide a time-efficient, publicly accessible means to allow international discussion among health care providers of clinically significant evidence-based research.[50] Social media have been shown to increase outreach from a scientific conference by increasing active participation. Web sites, such as Doximity, allow users to create an online presence and facilitate exchange of ideas and communication during the conference.[51]

Continuing medical education meetings
CME meetings are an invaluable resource for rheumatologists to keep abreast of the recent advances in rheumatology. In addition to disease-oriented topics, there has been an increased focus on quality improvement including aspects of performance improvement, patient outcomes, and community and public health issues.[52] Important CME meetings for rheumatologists include the ACR annual meeting, ACR Winter Rheumatology Symposium, and the ACR State-of-the-Art Clinical Symposium. There are many non-ACR CME meetings offered local to academic institutions as well as in big cities or resort areas. A few examples include the Congress of Clinical Rheumatology, Rheumatology Winter Clinical Symposium, Advances in Rheumatology, and Perspectives in Rheumatic Diseases. In-person CME conferences, while offering concentrated educational sessions predominately in lecture format and strong networking opportunities, impose the burden of travel costs and the cost to the practice of time away from the office and shot-term reduced patient access to care.

In recent years, efforts have been made to make conference content available online to better address individual physician schedule constraints and to allow physicians to learn at their own pace.[53] The ACR has initiated a streaming service, called "ACR Beyond," a subscription service providing high-quality educational presentations of scientific sessions and lectures that can be accessed globally via Internet connection. Online-based CME education is more cost-effective, and these programs have been found to be as effective in imparting knowledge as traditional CME formats.[54] Notably, the convenience of Internet access has limitations caused by lack of fixed time constraints and lack of pressure to complete the material, leading to non-completion of CME activities.[55]

Mechanisms to enhance the learning experience during CME activities have been introduced. Pretest and post-test questions are used to assess if the CME session learning objectives are achieved, providing invaluable input to faculty. Furthermore, involving pretest and post-test questions allows the educator to increase attention of the learners and encourage learners to seek information during the didactic lecture. Audience response systems (ARS) are electronic tools that allow groups of people to answer a question. Each person has a device in which selections can be made. The results are then polled and tabulated in real time and made available to participants.

The ARS provides learners with immediate and anonymous feedback regarding the accuracy of their responses. Audience response systems have been found effective in enhancing attention and improving enthusiasm and engagement among CME learners.[56] Crowdsourcing is an innovative instructional method, where ideas or content are obtained from contributions of large groups of people. A crowdsourcing discussion, based on problem-solving, may be an ideal way for adults to harness collective wisdom and expertise as a group.[57]

Industry-sponsored continuing medical education programs

Industry-sponsored CME programs have received significant attention within the medical community in recent years. Many CME activities are funded by industry. In 2014, 25% of the income reported by CME providers was industry sponsored.[58,59] Although these CME programs deliver updated information to providers regarding the latest treatments, research has shown that industry funding may skew CME content toward matching industry goals.[60] The health care industry and physicians have different fiduciary duties. Physicians have a fiduciary duty to do what is best for the patient while the health care companies' primary aims are to benefit their owners and shareholders.[61] Because of these ethical concerns, there has been a move away from reliance on industry support for CME programs in recent years. This of course creates a challenge in obtaining resources for programming given prior high reliance on this support.

Creative approaches are needed to ensure a productive and ethical relationship between physicians and pharmaceutical companies, such that medical education opportunities continue to be optimized. The rheumatologist should strive to be a conscientious learner at all times, critically analyzing the data presented, and demonstrating awareness for potential conflicts of interest. Even being a recipient of the smallest of gifts has been found to influence prescribing patterns.[62] Interventions aimed at educating the physician about conflict of interest, such as lectures with an evidence-based review and guidelines for conflict of interest, and teaching physicians to interact with industry representatives in a critical and inquisitive manner have been shown to be effective in changing physician perception and increasing awareness of the ethical concerns of gifts and industry-sponsored CME activities.[63–65]

Management of the relationships between physicians and industry refers to the way in which potentially harmful conflicts of interest are minimized while maintaining the relationships between these 2 entities.[66] Examples of management in CME include mandates by the ACCME that require CME program content be developed independent of the sponsor, requiring a preview of speakers' slides at CME events by CME committees, and diversification of industry sponsorship of activities (ie, not allowing any CME that is sponsored exclusively by a single pharmaceutical company).[66]

Maintenance of certification

Staying current with advances in medical knowledge is fundamental to lifelong learning. There are many mechanisms available, as already discussed, to maintain a physician's knowledge base. To demonstrate a physician's continued abilities in medical knowledge, skills, and attitudes, in this case for evaluating for or providing care to patients with rheumatic diseases, the ABIM has a Maintenance of Certification (MOC) program, and participation in MOC activities is requisite for staying board certified.[67] Rheumatologists who were ABIM certified prior to 1990 are "grandfathered or grandmothered," and these physicians are not required to participate in ABIM MOC activities in order to maintain board certification. If the grandfathered/grandmothered ABIM diplomates wish to demonstrate participation in ABIM MOC activities, they may enter one of two pathways for ABIM MOC. As of this writing, the ABIM reports board certification/recertification status of diplomates, and ABIM also reports whether a board-certified physician is participating in the MOC activities. In efforts to improve physician experience in participating in MOC activities, the ABIM has introduced a new option, a knowledge check-in, a shorter assessment taken every 2 years, that is lower stakes and open book. The 2-year assessments can be taken on one of several designated dates during the year, in the office or at home, to align with greater flexibility in scheduling given increasingly busy physician schedules. Alternatively, the secure 10-year examination is still offered as an MOC pathway, and it is now (as of 2019) also open book format. ABIM has included more options for earning MOC points for physicians including through participation in CME programs, manuscript reviews, reading in UpToDate for CME, and participating in practice improvement projects.[67] In addition to providing the CARE questions for MOC points, the ACR conducts MOC sessions during its annual meeting. Both of these learning opportunities provide valuable CME to physicians and help rheumatologists obtain MOC points needed for maintaining ABIM rheumatology board certification.

MEETING THE GOALS OF OPTIMIZING EDUCATION FOR PRACTICING RHEUMATOLOGISTS-RHEUMATOLOGY EDUCATION ACROSS THE AGES

In 1965, Lowell T. Coggeshall presented a report to the Association of American Medical Colleges entitled "Planning for Medical Progress through Education." In the report, he decried the stark separation that occurs between the 3 phases of physician education: medical school, graduate medical education, and CME, and recommended that medical education be planned and provided as a continuum.[68] Although delivering medical education as a continuum has not yet been achieved, recent progress has moved the field closer toward offering continuous rheumatology education for rheumatologists across the ages.

The evolution of competency-based medical education from the traditional medical education model is one of the key steps toward offering continuous rheumatology education for rheumatologists across the ages. In the traditional model, educational objectives and assessment were established based on a curriculum. However, in competency-based medical education, the needs of the population and health systems are first assessed. Based on these needs, core competencies are developed. The core competencies form the foundation of both the curriculum and the assessment. Because the traditional model of medical education is curricular-based, it is teacher-centered and displays rigidity based on the learner having to perform specific activities for a specific amount of time. Competency-based medical education differs in that it is learner-centered, and its design is based on competencies. The learner may thus advance at different rates based on aptitude. Milestones have been developed to allow monitoring of the learner's mastery in competency-based medical education. Milestones are observable developmental steps demonstrating increasing levels of competence and are organized under the 6 domains of ACGME core competencies (see **Box 1**). Entrustable professional activities (EPAs) are routine professional life activities of physicians specific to a subspecialty.[69] EPAs reflect the actions, knowledge, skills, and attitudes that define the specialty; the fellow who has achieved competency in each of the 14 rheumatology EPAs is ready for unsupervised practice.[70] Each practicing rheumatologist, likewise, has accomplished and continues to demonstrate competence in each of the rheumatology EPAs.

Defining and providing a continuum in learning for the rheumatologist across the span of a career is not only a challenge but should be an aspiration as one considers the ongoing evolution of rheumatology education. The scientific innovations in this field and the expanding access to learning activities afforded by technology intercalate to enrich lifelong learning.

THE FUTURE OF MEDICAL EDUCATION FOR THE RHEUMATOLOGIST

The authors believe that significant progress has been made regarding optimizing rheumatologists' education. The future for learning across the continuum of a career promises opportunity and innovation. Although many challenges for the rheumatology workforce are predicted, there is great security and promise for the diversity of learning activities availed to all rheumatology care providers. Because it is in physician's best interest to continue to produce generations of capable rheumatologists, medical education must continue to be prioritized with sufficient resources appropriated. There are many important stakeholders for rheumatology education, including patients, rheumatologists, rheumatology nurse practitioners and physician assistants, colleagues and referring providers, medical students, internal medicine residents, rheumatology fellows, rheumatology societies, industry, academic institutions, and the federal government. Strong leadership and effective strategic planning involving all stakeholders with a common vision for the future of rheumatology education are important. Hopefully, this will lead to a concerted, organized approach toward medical education of rheumatologists. By putting population needs and learners' needs at the center, the path to defining and providing high value, easily accessible, technologically innovative, and engaging educational activities will be facilitated. Scientific discovery relies on and invites learning, and this specialty is thus well-situated to further explore and accomplish learning across the continuum of a rheumatology career.

SUMMARY

A multifaceted approach is warranted to optimize medical education for rheumatologists across the career span. Medical education for rheumatologists in the future has to involve all stages in the development of a well-trained rheumatologist-readying the fellow for practice, effectively transitioning from fellowship to practice, and promoting lifelong learning in rheumatology. These efforts should be based on adult learning theory to enhance learning, and ACGME core competencies, milestones, and entrustable professional activities for standardization. It is also critical to provide sufficient breadth in content to accommodate differing career pathways. Efforts should be made to leverage advances in information technology and deliver content through different avenues to ensure education is accessible to all rheumatologists who may have diverse lifestyles, practice/working patterns, and family obligations. This is particularly important going forward in view of the changing demographics of the rheumatology workforce: increased number of part-time practitioners, increased attention being placed on lifestyle, and increased rate of retirement of current rheumatologists.[4] There has been significant progress, and all stakeholders including rheumatologists themselves, should continue to take a proactive approach to optimize education as practitioners strive to maintain the strongest and most accessible rheumatology work force.

REFERENCES

1. Battafarano DF, Ditmyer M, Bolster MB, et al. 2015 American college of rheumatology workforce study: supply and demand projections of adult rheumatology workforce, 2015-2030. Arthritis Care Res (Hoboken) 2018;70(4):617–26.

2. Yazdany J, MacLean CH. Quality of care in the rheumatic diseases: current status and future directions. Curr Opin Rheumatol 2008;20(2):159–66.
3. Woolf AD. Specialist training in rheumatology in Europe. Rheumatology (Oxford) 2002;41(9):1062–6.
4. Bolster MB, Bass AR, Hausmann JS, et al. 2015 American college of rheumatology workforce study: the role of graduate medical education in adult rheumatology. Arthritis Rheumatol 2018;70(6):817–25.
5. Research AIf. Adult learning theories. 2011. Available at: https://lincs.ed.gov/state-resources/federal-initiatives/teal/guide/adultlearning. Accessed October 7, 2018.
6. Cooper AZ, Richards JB. Lectures for adult learners: breaking old habits in graduate medical education. Am J Med 2017;130(3):376–81.
7. Taylor DC, Hamdy H. Adult learning theories: implications for learning and teaching in medical education: AMEE Guide No. 83. Med Teach 2013;35(11):e1561–72.
8. Patwardhan A, Henrickson M, Laskosz L, et al. Current pediatric rheumatology fellowship training in the United States: what fellows actually do. Pediatr Rheumatol Online J 2014;12:8.
9. American College of Rheumatology. Core curriculum outline for rheumatology fellowship programs. 2015.Available at: https://www.rheumatology.org/Portals/0/Files/Core%20Curriculum%20Outline_2015.pdf. Accessed October 7, 2018.
10. Criscione-Schreiber LG, Brown CR Jr, O'Rourke KS, et al. New roadmap for the journey from internist to rheumatologist. Arthritis Care Res (Hoboken) 2017;69(6):769–75.
11. American College of Rheumatology. Rheum4Science Module 1 - Overview of innate immunity. 2018. Available at: https://www.rheumatology.org/Learning-Center/Educational-Activities/View/ID/881. Accessed October 7, 2018.
12. American College of Rheumatology. Adult rheumatology in-training examination. 2018. Available at: https://www.rheumatology.org/Learning-Center/Academic-Resources/Adult-in-Training-Exam.
13. Lohr KM, Clauser A, Hess BJ, et al. Performance on the adult rheumatology in-training examination and relationship to outcomes on the rheumatology certification examination. Arthritis Rheumatol 2015;67(11):3082–90.
14. American Board of Internal Medicine. Rheumatology certification examination blueprint. 2018. Available at: https://www.abim.org/~/media/ABIM%20Public/Files/pdf/exam-blueprints/certification/rheumatology.pdf. Accessed August 25, 2018.
15. Torralba KD, Cannella AC, Kissin EY, et al. Musculoskeletal ultrasound instruction in adult rheumatology fellowship programs. Arthritis Care Res (Hoboken) 2017. [Epub ahead of print].
16. Samuels J, Abramson SB, Kaeley GS. The use of musculoskeletal ultrasound by rheumatologists in the United States. Bull NYU Hosp Jt Dis 2010;68(4):292–8.
17. Ultrasound School of North American Rheumatologists. Ultrasound School of North American Rheumatologists-training program. Available at: www.ussonar.org/training/overview/. Accessed, 2018.
18. American College of Rheumatology. RhMSUS Certification. 2018. Available at: https://www.rheumatology.org/Learning-Center/RhMSUS-Certification.
19. Lewiecki EM, Binkley N, Morgan SL, et al. Best Practices for dual-energy x-ray absorptiometry measurement and reporting: international society for clinical densitometry guidance. J Clin Densitom 2016;19(2):127–40.
20. Weiner JJ, Eudy AM, Criscione-Schreiber LG. How well do rheumatology fellows manage acute infusion reactions? a pilot curricular intervention. Arthritis Care Res (Hoboken) 2018;70(6):931–7.

21. Ancowitz B, Shah SA. Infusion services in the gastroenterology practice. Gastrointest Endosc Clin N Am 2006;16(4):727–42.

22. The Rheumatologist. Managing an In-Office Infusion Practice. 2012. Available at: https://www.the-rheumatologist.org/article/managing-an-in-office-infusion-practice/. Accessed, 2018.

23. Wichman CL, Netzel PJ, Menaker R. Preparing psychiatric residents for the "real world": a practice management curriculum. Acad Psychiatry 2009;33(2):131–4.

24. Falvo T, McKniff S, Smolin G, et al. The business of emergency medicine: a nonclinical curriculum proposal for emergency medicine residency programs. Acad Emerg Med 2009;16(9):900–7.

25. Gunderman RB, Tawadros AM. Business education for radiology residents the value of full-time business educators. Acad Radiol 2011;18(5):645–9.

26. Holak EJ, Kaslow O, Pagel PS. Facilitating the transition to practice: a weekend retreat curriculum for business-of-medicine education of United States anesthesiology residents. J Anesth 2010;24(5):807–10.

27. American College of Rheumatology. Practice Publications. 2018. Available at: https://www.rheumatology.org/Practice-Quality/Administrative-Support/Practice-Resources/Practice-Publications.

28. American College of Rheumatology. Tools & training from the American College of Rheumatology Practice Management Team. The Rheumatologist 2018.

29. Medical Group Management Association. Body of knowledge. Available at: https://www.mgma.com/career-pathways/career-advancement/board-certification/board-certification-requirements/body-of-knowledge. Accessed August 28, 2018.

30. Backer LA. Back to school: options for learning the business of medicine. Fam Pract Manag 2001;8(7):27–33.

31. American Academy of Family Physicians. Basics of quality improvement. Available at: https://www.aafp.org/practice-management/improvement/basics.html. Accessed August 26, 2018.

32. Prince LK, Little DJ, Schexneider KI, et al. Integrating quality improvement education into the nephrology curricular milestones framework and the clinical learning environment review. Clin J Am Soc Nephrol 2017;12(2):349–56.

33. Chew LD, Watanabe JM, Buchwald D, et al. Junior faculty's perspectives on mentoring. Acad Med 2003;78(6):652.

34. Carole B, Anne T, Sindie S. Feature: mentoring systems: benefits and challenges of diverse mentoring partnerships. 2018. Available at: https://www.aamc.org/members/gfa/faculty_vitae/146014/mentoring_systems.html.

35. Davidson A, Polsky D. Sustaining the rheumatology research enterprise. Arthritis Care Res (Hoboken) 2015;67(9):1187–90.

36. Nigrovic PA, Muscal E, Riebschleger M, et al. AMIGO: a novel approach to the mentorship gap in pediatric rheumatology. J Pediatr 2014;164(2):226–7.e1-3.

37. Mehta SJ, Forde KA. How to make a successful transition from fellowship to faculty in an academic medical center. Gastroenterology 2013;145(4):703–7.

38. Anwar H, Batty H. Continuing medical education strategy for primary health care physicians in Oman: lessons to be learnt. Oman Med J 2007;22(3):33–5.

39. National Center for Biotechnology Information. U.S National Library of Medicine. PubMed Central. Available at: https://www.ncbi.nlm.nih.gov/pmc/.

40. Kwag KH, Gonzalez-Lorenzo M, Banzi R, et al. Providing doctors with high-quality information: an updated evaluation of web-based point-of-care information summaries. J Med Internet Res 2016;18(1):e15.

41. Moja L, Banzi R. Navigators for medicine: evolution of online point-of-care evidence-based services. Int J Clin Pract 2011;65(1):6–11.

42. Wikipedia. Social media. 2018. Available at: https://en.wikipedia.org/wiki/Social_media.

43. Vohra RS, Hallissey MT. Social networks, social media, and innovating surgical education. JAMA Surg 2015;150(3):192–3.

44. Dyson MP, Newton AS, Shave K, et al. Social media for the dissemination of Cochrane child health evidence: evaluation study. J Med Internet Res 2017;19(9): e308.

45. Gates A, Featherstone R, Shave K, et al. Dissemination of evidence in paediatric emergency medicine: a quantitative descriptive evaluation of a 16-week social media promotion. BMJ Open 2018;8(6):e022298.

46. Buckarma EH, Thiels CA, Gas BL, et al. Influence of social media on the dissemination of a traditional surgical research article. J Surg Educ 2017;74(1):79–83.

47. Sinha MS, Freifeld CC, Brownstein JS, et al. Social media impact of the Food and Drug Administration's drug safety communication messaging about zolpidem: mixed-methods analysis. JMIR Public Health Surveill 2018;4(1):e1.

48. Flynn S, Hebert P, Korenstein D, et al. Leveraging social media to promote evidence-based continuing medical education. PLoS One 2017;12(1):e0168962.

49. Goff D, Jones C, Toney B, et al. Use of twitter to educate and engage surgeons in infectious diseases and antimicrobial stewardship. Infect Dis Clin Pract 2016; 24(6):324–7.

50. Roberts MJ, Perera M, Lawrentschuk N, et al. Globalization of continuing professional development by journal clubs via microblogging: a systematic review. J Med Internet Res 2015;17(4):e103.

51. Chan WS, Leung AY. Use of social network sites for communication among health professionals: systematic review. J Med Internet Res 2018;20(3):e117.

52. Balmer JT. The transformation of continuing medical education (CME) in the United States. Adv Med Educ Pract 2013;4:171–82.

53. Wiecha J, Barrie N. Collaborative online learning: a new approach to distance CME. Acad Med 2002;77(9):928–9.

54. Wutoh R, Boren SA, Balas EA. eLearning: a review of Internet-based continuing medical education. J Contin Educ Health Prof 2004;24(1):20–30.

55. Keis O, Grab C, Schneider A, et al. Online or face-to-face instruction? A qualitative study on the electrocardiogram course at the University of Ulm to examine why students choose a particular format. BMC Med Educ 2017;17(1):194.

56. Miller RG, Ashar BH, Getz KJ. Evaluation of an audience response system for the continuing education of health professionals. J Contin Educ Health Prof 2003; 23(2):109–15.

57. Penciner R. Crowdsourcing: an instructional method at an emergency medicine continuing education course. CJEM 2015;17(4):433–6.

58. Accreditation Council for Continuing Medical Education. Accreditation Council for Continuing Medical Education annual report 2014. 2014. Available at: http://www.accme.org/sites/default/files/630_20150707_2014_Annual_Report.pdf. Accessed October 7, 2018.

59. American Board of Internal Medicine. Maintenance of Certification (MOC). Available at: https://www.abim.org/maintenance-of-certification/default.aspx. Accessed August 28, 2018.

60. Davis DA. CME and the pharmaceutical industry: two worlds, three views, four steps. CMAJ 2004;171(2):149–50.

61. Board ESC. The future of continuing medical education: the roles of medical professional societies and the health care industry: Position paper prepared with contributions from the European Society of Cardiology Committees for Advocacy,

Education and Industry Relations, Endorsed by the Board of the European Society of Cardiology. Eur Heart J 2018. [Epub ahead of print].

62. King M, Bearman PS. Gifts and influence: conflict of interest policies and prescribing of psychotropic medications in the United States. Soc Sci Med 2017; 172:153–62.

63. Agrawal S, Saluja I, Kaczorowski J. A prospective before-and-after trial of an educational intervention about pharmaceutical marketing. Acad Med 2004; 79(11):1046–50.

64. Schneider JA, Arora V, Kasza K, et al. Residents' perceptions over time of pharmaceutical industry interactions and gifts and the effect of an educational intervention. Acad Med 2006;81(7):595–602.

65. Wilkes MS, Hoffman JR. An innovative approach to educating medical students about pharmaceutical promotion. Acad Med 2001;76(12):1271–7.

66. Raad R, Appelbaum PS. Relationships between medicine and industry: approaches to the problem of conflicts of interest. Annu Rev Med 2012;63:465–77.

67. American Board of Internal Medicine. MOC assessments in 2018. Available at: https://www.abim.org/maintenance-of-certification/moc-requirements/general.aspx.

68. Aschenbrener CA, Ast C, Kirch DG. Graduate medical education: its role in achieving a true medical education continuum. Acad Med 2015;90(9):1203–9.

69. Brown CR Jr, Criscione-Schreiber L, O'Rourke KS, et al. What is a rheumatologist and how do we make one? Arthritis Care Res (Hoboken) 2016;68(8):1166–72.

70. American College of Rheumatology. Adult Rheumatology Entrustable Professional Activities (EPA). 2018. Available at: https://www.rheumatology.org/Portals/0/Files/Adult%20Rheumatology%20EPAs.pdf.

The Challenges of Approaching and Managing Gout

Theodore R. Fields, MD

KEYWORDS

• Gout • Gouty arthritis • Patient education • Physician education

KEY POINTS

- Despite excellent therapies, most patients with gout are not adequately managed, and patients and providers have many misconceptions about gout.
- Patient education and monitoring are critical to optimal gout outcomes, and rheumatologists in various practice settings can use the modalities, individuals, and teams that best suit their resources and patient population.
- Newer FDA-approved urate-lowering agents (febuxostat, pegloticase, and lesinurad) offer alternatives to allopurinol in appropriate settings.
- Pipeline medications, such as arhalofenate and canakinumab, may provide future additional options in gout management.

INTRODUCTION

Improving the care of patients with gout is an important national health priority. Gouty arthritis is an important quality of life and economic issue. In the United States, there are an estimated 8.3 million patients with gout, a 3.9% prevalence.[1] The costs of gout to society are high.[2] Multiple studies reflect the effect of gout on quality of life[3,4] and its association with an increased mortality.[5] Although the hospitalization rate has been dropping in patients with rheumatoid arthritis, it is increasing in gout.[6] Gout is associated with kidney stones, and travels with many comorbidities.[7]

Therapy for gout is effective, yet most patients with gout do not reach their urate goal.[8–10] Many reasons have been postulated for this failure, including patient misconceptions,[11] nonadherence to medication,[12] and comorbidities crowding out time for gout discussion at physician visits.[7] **Box 1** lists some postulated major reasons for the high degree of nonadherence to urate-lowering therapy (ULT).

Disclosure Statement: Advisory Board: Takeda Pharmaceuticals, Horizon Pharmaceuticals. Advisory Board and Speakers' Bureau: Ironwood Pharmaceuticals.
Division of Rheumatology, Hospital for Special Surgery, 535 East 70th Street, Suite 848G, New York, NY 10021, USA
E-mail address: fieldst@hss.edu

Rheum Dis Clin N Am 45 (2019) 145–157
https://doi.org/10.1016/j.rdc.2018.09.009
0889-857X/19/

> **Box 1**
> **Why do people with gout not take their urate-lowering medication?**
>
> - They feel better between flares and stop treatment
> - They do not understand that gout is "still there" between episodes
> - They do not believe that they can become "gout-free" if they stay with the medication; they often think that having gout flares is part of the immutable long-term picture
> - They have many comorbidities and thus many medications, and do not want more
> - They think diet is the answer, but they just have not done it well enough; they think it is "their fault," even after being educated about gout's genetic basis
> - Mobilization flares when starting urate-lowering therapy make them lose confidence in treatment effectiveness, and they abandon urate-lowering therapy

Rheumatologists see patients in many settings: small private practice, group practice, community hospital, academic practice, and settings focused on care of the elderly. Many approaches have been examined for addressing unmet needs of patients with gout, focusing especially on patient education and monitoring, and their use varies depending on size and setting of rheumatology practices. Many of these strategies also are likely effective in internal medicine practices.

Guidelines[13,14] agree that once the diagnosis of gout is established, the need for lifelong therapy is needed, and in most cases diet and lifestyle change is insufficient. This requires that physicians caring for patients with gout need to go beyond initial appropriate prescribing and motivate patients toward long-term adherence and find ways to appropriately monitor that adherence. Several tools have been developed to assist in these efforts.

CHALLENGES IN DIAGNOSING GOUT

The diagnosis of gout is often straightforward in patients with classic presentations. However, there continue to be patients diagnosed with gout who actually have pseudogout, Lyme disease, or other conditions. There are also patients with gout who are given incorrect diagnoses, such as rheumatoid arthritis. Many diagnostic and classification algorithms have been published for gout. The 2015 Gout Classification Criteria, a combined American College of Rheumatology (ACR) and European League Against Rheumatism effort, is probably the most useful produced to date.[15] **Table 1** provides a review of these criteria. Classification criteria are designed to identify homogeneous populations for studies, but highly descriptive classification criteria such as these are useful in diagnosis. This set of criteria requires 8 points for gout classification, based on classic features, such as intense and intermittent episodes, and involvement of typical locations, such as the first metatarsophalangeal joint. These classification criteria can be calculated online at http://goutclassificationcalculator.auckland.ac.nz/. In a patient with a finger lesion as shown in **Figure 1**, where there was no prior history suggestive of gout, the white deposits on the distal interphalangeal joint (see **Fig. 1**A) proved to be monosodium urate crystals (see **Fig. 1**B) via polarizing microscopy, confirming tophaceous gout. Once crystals are identified, the patient is classified as having gout without needing additional criteria other than having had at least one episode of swelling, pain, or tenderness in a peripheral joint or bursa. There are no specific exclusion criteria in this classification scheme, because gout can coexist with other conditions. Patients with classic tophi, such as demonstrated in **Fig. 2**, get 4 points toward being classified as gout and with elevated serum

Table 1 Gout classification scoring			
Clinical Domains	First MTP monoarticular or oligoarticular = 2 points
	Ankle/midfoot monoarticular or oligoarticular = 1 point
Domain 1: joint involvement	Other pattern = 0 points
	MAX = 2 points
Domain 2: episode characteristics	Erythema over joint = 1 point
	Cannot bear touch to joint = 1 point
	Difficulty walking/using joint = 1 point
	MAX = 3 points
Domain 3: time course of episodes	
Time to maximal pain <24 h	2 or more episodes with 2 or more qualities = 2 points
Time to resolution <14 d	1 episode with 2 or more qualities = 1 point
Resolution between episodes	MAX = 2 points
Domain 4: tophus	Clinical evidence of tophus 4 points, none = 0 points
Laboratory domains	Positive crystals = proven gout
Monosodium urate crystal identification	Negative aspirate for crystals = -2 points
	MAX = 0 points
Serum urate	>10 = 4 points
	8–10 = 3 points
	6–8 = 2 points
	4–6 = 0 points
	<4 = -4 points
	MAX = 4 points
Imaging domains	US or DECT evidence of urate deposition = 4 points
Urate deposition US or DECT	No evidence on US or DECT = 0 points
	MAX = 4 points
Gouty erosion	Gouty erosion hands[a] and/or feet on radiograph = 4 points
	No evidence = 0 points
	MAX = 4 points

Note: If urate crystals are demonstrated under polarizing microscopy, this suffices for classification of gout. Without crystal identification, 8 points required for classification.

Abbreviations: DECT, dual-energy computed tomography scan; MAX, maximum; MTP, metatarsophalangeal joint; US, ultrasound.

[a] Exclude DIP joint.

Adapted from Neogi T, Jansen TL, Dalbeth N, et al. 2015 gout classification criteria: an American College of Rheumatology/European League Against Rheumatism collaborative initiative. Ann Rheum Dis 2015;74:1789–98; with permission.

urate (SUA) likely meet gout classification criteria without the need for microscopic crystal identification. In less typical cases, crystal identification is often required.

GOUT CARE HAS BEEN SUBOPTIMAL NATIONALLY AND INTERNATIONALLY

Improvements in gout management are clearly needed. Despite numerous widely accepted guidelines proposing a treat-to-target strategy,[13,14,16] the evidence for low medication adherence and failure to reach therapeutic urate goals for patients with gout is overwhelming.

Patients with gout have been shown to have several specific knowledge gaps in several studies, and harbor stereotypes about patients with gout that are not helpful.[11,17,18] **Box 2** reviews what these studies have found to be among the most

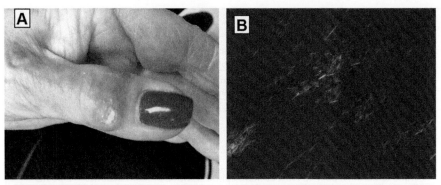

Fig. 1. Microscopic demonstration of tophaceous material. (*A*) Image of patient's thumb interphalangeal joint with whitish material with surrounding erythema, with no history of gout. (*B*) Image of polarizing microscopic view of material from surface of thumb interphalangeal joint showing negatively birefringent monosodium urate crystals diagnostic of gout.

common of these gaps and misconceptions. As a result of lack of information, or faulty information, patients often fail to start or continue ULT, along with blaming themselves for their continued gout flares.

THE PREVALENCE OF GOUT IS RISING, WITH UNMET NEEDS

The incidence of gout has more than doubled over the past 20 years. This increase together with the more frequent occurrence of comorbid conditions and cardiovascular risk factors represents a significant public health challenge.[7]

The suboptimal care of gout internationally needs a multifaceted approach. Patient education, as the cornerstone to medication adherence, is a key factor. **Box 1** reviews many of the reasons patients with gout stop, or do not start, ULT. **Box 2** reviews important knowledge gaps that prevent patients from having needed discussions with their physician and cause them to avoid or abandon ULT.

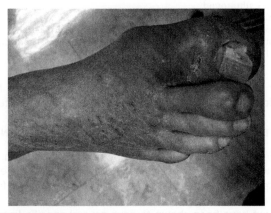

Fig. 2. Classic tophi. This patient has classic appearance of tophi, including irregular shape, whitish material seen under the skin of the distal second toe, and first toe shows overlying increased vascularity.

> **Box 2**
> **What are some of the things most poorly understood by patients with gout?**
>
> - Not understanding the importance of lowering urate level
> - Not knowing their urate goal
> - Not appreciating the concept of mobilization flares or the need for bridge therapy when starting ULT
> - Not appreciating the genetic aspect of gout
> - Not appreciating the limited ability of diet alone to allow them to achieve urate goal
> - Harboring stereotypes of patients with gout as overweight drinkers, leading to self-blame and focus on diet to the exclusion of ULT

PRINCIPLES OF GOUT MANAGEMENT

Many guidelines have been published regarding gout management. The most extensive and detailed of these are the ACR 2012 guidelines.[13,19] All published guidelines, with one exception,[20] advise treating gout to a specific urate level (treat-to-target). The ACR guidelines propose treating all patients with gout to less than 6.0, and those with tophi to less than 5.0. Although further randomized, double-blind controlled studies will be helpful, the literature strongly supports treating a urate goal by demonstrating reduced flares of gout with lower urate levels.[21–23] Present guidelines to not propose treatment of asymptomatic hyperuricemia, and data so far have not been adequate for Food and Drug Administration (FDA) approval of urate lowering for renal or cardiovascular benefits.

There has been debate about how low to aim with ULT in difficult patients with gout, such as those with multiple tophi. Perez-Ruiz and coworkers[24] has shown that tophi shrink more rapidly when urate levels are lower and pegloticase studies have shown rapid reduction in tophi with dramatic reductions in SUA.[25] However, the potential of low SUA to potentiate neurodegenerative conditions, such as Parkinson disease,[26] although controversial, led the 2016 European League Against Rheumatism gout guidelines to recommend against lowering continuously the SUA level to less than 3 mg/dL in the long term, that is, for several years.[14] The 2012 ACR guidelines do not address the degree of SUA lowering beyond saying that "the target SUA should be lowered sufficiently to durably improve signs and symptoms of gout, including palpable and visible tophi" and that this may involve therapeutic SUA level lowering to less than 5 mg/dL.[15]

Acute management of gout includes colchicine, nonsteroidal anti-inflammatory drugs (NSAIDs), and oral or injected corticosteroids. In patients who fail or are contraindicated for all of these, anakinra has been shown to be effective, consistent with the interleukin (IL)-1β prominence in gout flare pathophysiology.[27,28] Chronic urate lowering is attained first line with xanthine oxidase inhibitors (XOI), and if the patient fails to achieve urate goal a uricosuric agent is added. In refractory cases, intravenous pegloticase is used. When any ULT is started, it is advised to concomitantly start gout flare prophylaxis, most commonly with colchicine, but also low-dose NSAIDs or prednisone is used. Allopurinol is the most commonly used first-line agent, and ACR guidelines advised to start at 100 mg daily[13] and increase at 2- to 5-week intervals until the monosodium urate goal is achieved. For patients with Han Chinese or Thai backgrounds, or Korean background with estimated glomerular filtration rate (eGFR) less than 60, ACR guidelines advise checking the HLA-B*5801 genetic marker before starting allopurinol, because this marker is associated with a markedly increased risk of severe allopurinol hypersensitivity reaction. African Americans also have a high incidence of this marker, and it also may be reasonable to consider checking the HLA-B*5801 marker in this group.[29]

Febuxostat is an XOI available as an alternative to allopurinol. It has the advantage of only 3% renal excretion. The CARES study looked at the relative cardiovascular safety of allopurinol versus febuxostat and raised more questions than answers.[30] Taken together, the cardiovascular MACE criteria (myocardial infarction, stroke, cardiovascular death, and urgent need for revascularization) had similar outcomes with allopurinol and febuxostat. However, in secondary outcome evaluation cardiovascular death was statistically significantly higher with febuxostat. Complicating interpretation were a large number of dropouts in the study and the finding that most deaths in the study came after the patients had stopped taking their XOI, be it allopurinol or febuxostat. Choi and colleagues,[31] discussed the potential relevance of the CARES study, and the associated FDA public safety alert, to the prescribing patterns of ULT. The authors question whether febuxostat should be considered as a first-line agent. Some have considered febuxostat as a first-line ULT in patients with reduced renal function, in view of its low renal clearance and ability to use unchanged dosing in patients with eGFR from 30 mL/min to 60 mL/min. The authors point out that it has been shown to be safe to raise allopurinol doses (slowly) in patients with decreased renal function.[32] Some have also suggested that febuxostat may have an advantage in patients with renal insufficiency because those patients are at higher risk of allopurinol hypersensitivity syndrome. Choi and colleagues[31] cite data on the ability to reduce this risk by starting at low allopurinol doses and increasing slowly, along with addressing other risk factors for allopurinol hypersensitivity, such as the presence of the HLA B*5801 genetic marker as discussed previously.[33] For patients with gout with a prior history of cardiovascular disease who are doing well with and tolerating febuxostat, discussing the CARES data and shared decision making with each patient seems prudent.

Probenecid is a uricosuric agent that is added to XOI therapy, but it requires a twice daily dosing regimen and has had some tolerability issues including nausea and lightheadedness. More recently, lesinurad has been introduced, which is given along with an XOI. A combination pill combining lesinurad with allopurinol is available. Creatinine elevations with lesinurad have been noted, but 89% of increases of 1.5 to 2 × baseline creatinine level were reversible, and 100% of creatinine level increases greater than 2.0 × baseline were reversible. With the 200-mg dose of lesinurad, the FDA-approved dose, no renal failure was reported in these studies.[34,35]

When patients are refractory to other ULT options, intravenous pegloticase is used. This agent often brings SUA to undetectable levels and has been associated with rapid improvement in tophi and with fewer gout flares after 3 months of therapy.[23,25] Checking SUA before each infusion and stopping infusions for patients where the SUA is greater than 6.0 has been shown to markedly reduce the risk of infusion reactions.[36]

When starting any ULT, guidelines advise the use of bridge therapy, usually 6 months, to help prevent the early flares that can result from urate mobilization. Colchicine has been most studied in this regard[37] but in some settings low-dose NSAIDs or steroids have been used.

Despite optimal use of the armamentarium of available gout therapy, adherence issues often lead to failure of gout management. Significant efforts to improve adherence seem likely to make a major difference in gout outcomes, and are described next.

SPECIAL POPULATIONS IN GOUT MANAGEMENT

Renal disease has been a barrier to effective management of gout. Abnormal renal function is associated with an increased risk of the allopurinol hypersensitivity syndrome. Issues related to allopurinol dosing in renal insufficiency and strategies for reducing the risk of allopurinol hypersensitivity are discussed previously in the section on febuxostat.

Cardiovascular disease is important in gout because it is known that patients with gout are at higher cardiovascular risk.[7] Some medications for acute gout, such as NSAIDs and prednisone, may be problematic in patients with congestive heart failure. In the hospital, clinicians may need to turn to anakinra[27] therapy to avoid fluid retention in heart failure patients with gout flares. A recent article on cardiovascular safety of febuxostat versus allopurinol is discussed previously.[30]

Elderly patients with gout often have decreased eGFR, making NSAIDs for acute flares problematic. Other comorbidities, such as diabetes and hypertension, likewise need consideration in gout medication choice. Cognitive issues may make education and monitoring more difficult. Elderly patients are often on multiple medications that may have interactions with colchicine. Amiodarone raises colchicine levels, as do most statin drugs (but not rosuvastatin), and the greatest increases of colchicine levels are seen with cyclosporine and clarithromycin (colchicine package insert https://general.takedapharm.com/COLCRYSPI).

SETTING OF GOUT CARE: SPECIAL CIRCUMSTANCES

Care of patients with gout in the hospital has been shown to need improvement. A study of hospitalized patients with gout showed that many had nothing noted in their discharge plans regarding long-term ULT, although this was less of an issue when the rheumatology service consulted.[38] With the multiple issues being address in the hospital, gout flare can end up being treated as an episodic issue, without addressing long-term management. Patients in skilled nursing facilities have the special issues of the elderly described previously.

WHICH GROUPS OF PROFESSIONALS CAN HELP THE PHYSICIAN IMPROVE GOUT CARE?

Because education and monitoring are so crucial for gout patient medication adherence, researchers have looked at nurses and pharmacists as potential solutions.

Nurses have been used in studies of gout patient education and monitoring.[39] Pharmacist-run programs including algorithms for dose adjustment have been done[40,41] with results less impressive than in the nurse-run programs. A multidisciplinary team approach with nursing education and pharmacist monitoring has been tried, which also included a social worker to help patients overcome financial, language/cultural, and health literacy barriers to care.[17] This pilot study found that this multidisciplinary approach was feasible for settings where such a team was available, and suggested further evaluation of this strategy.

WHAT OTHER STRATEGIES HAVE BEEN TRIED FOR GOUT PATIENT EDUCATION?

Monitoring of gout patient adherence to medication has been done by telephone[17,41] and other options include text messaging and messaging within the patient portal of an electronic medical record. The goal of the initial gout patient educational intervention is to move them in the direction of self-management, and helping them form a long-term plan that they can follow.[42] Repeat educational interventions seem to be helpful in maintaining patient knowledge level[43] and formal self-management knowledge level examinations have been used to evaluate and then guide focused instruction to patients with gout.[11,17,44] Online resources for patients with gout are numerous, including: the Gout & Uric Acid Education Society (http://gouteducation.org/), the ACR (https://www.rheumatology.org/I-Am-A/Patient-Caregiver/Diseases-Conditions/Gout), Hospital for Special Surgery (https://www.hss.edu/conditions_gout-risk-factors-diagnosis-treatment.asp), and the CreakyJoints patient guideline for gout (https://creakyjoints.org/education/gout-patient-guidelines/).

HOW CAN RHEUMATOLOGISTS IN DIFFERENT PRACTICE SETTINGS BEST MANAGE PATIENTS WITH GOUT OVER TIME?

Each practice setting has different resources to mobilize for gout patient education and monitoring. **Box 3** provides a summary of possible options in different practice settings. For rheumatologists, optimum gout management also includes education of primary care physicians, because they manage the bulk of gout cases.

If resources are limited, consideration can be given to strategies to identify patients at highest risk of nonadherence. Questionnaires can be given to patients at the beginning of ULT[11,17,44] to identify patients with the largest knowledge gaps. These patients can be targeted for further specific education and monitoring, such as with scripted curriculum reviewed by a nurse and/or with follow-up calls or text messages to encourage adherence.

Box 3
Strategies for gout management in different rheumatology practice settings

- Small practice
  - Nurse/nurse practitioner/physician assistant most likely as educator and monitor of adherence to therapy
  - Nurse practitioner or physician assistant can follow algorithm and manage ULT titration
  - Consider text-messaging or telephone monitoring of adherence versus electronic medical record messaging
  - Consider such strategies as questionnaires, to identify patients least likely to adhere to regimen

- Group multispecialty practice that includes a rheumatologist
  - Nurse/nurse practitioner/physician assistant most likely, but could consider hiring pharmacist; could consider multidisciplinary approach
  - Consider text-messaging or telephone monitoring of adherence versus electronic medical record messaging
  - Rheumatologist educates internists (to treat-to-target and about importance of educating patients with gout) and is available for refractory cases

- Large academic practice
  - Pharmacist or nurse patient education, or team approach including social worker
  - Pharmacist or nurse monitoring (text/email or telephone, electronic medical record messaging)
  - Pharmacist can use algorithm for dose adjustment
  - Patient support groups and/or community programs
  - Consider text-messaging or telephone monitoring of adherence

- Skilled nursing facility or outpatient practice focused on elderly
  - Pharmacist or nurse educator skilled in special problems with hearing/memory
  - Closer monitoring regarding changes in eGFR and compliance
  - Monitoring for infection masquerading as gout flare

- Consultation service seeing in-patient gout
  - At discharge, have ULT plan in discharge summary
  - If volume sufficient, train nurse for postdischarge education

WHAT ARE PIPELINE DEVELOPMENTS IN GOUT THAT MAY HAVE AN EFFECT ON FUTURE MANAGEMENT?

Arhalofenate is uricosuric and seems to also have effectiveness against gouty inflammation. This agent is a peroxisome proliferator-activated receptor-γ partial agonist, which can lower urate and also inhibits expression of IL-1β. Arhalofenate was compared with allopurinol and placebo, and although not superior to allopurinol it did demonstrate a dual action of urate-lowering and anti-inflammatory effect.[45] Further study is needed but the use of a dual-action agent, which can lower urate and prevent early mobilization flares, could potentially avoid the need to start a "bridge" agent, such as colchicine, when ULT is started. Patients with gout are often resistant to starting one agent to lower urate, and especially resistant to adding the bridge medication. Having one agent with both actions could improve adherence.

Anakinra has been used off-label for years in refractory gout or in patients with contraindication to other available gout treatments.[27,28] It has not to date been approved by the FDA for this indication. There are settings, especially in hospitalized patients, where corticosteroids, NSAIDs, and colchicine are all contraindicated, and anakinra seems to have a role. Patients with renal dysfunction, diabetes, and congestive heart failure have decreased therapeutic options for gout flares. There are specific similar outpatient situations where this medication may also potentially benefit the patient.

Canakinumab, as a long-acting inhibitor of IL1-β, has potential to work as a bridge agent in patients who cannot take medications, such as colchicine or NSAIDs, when they are starting ULT, and might be considered as acute gout therapy. Studies of canakinumab showed efficacy in both these settings,[46,47] but the FDA has not approved it. The European Medicines Agency, however, has approved it. There are patients with gout who get recurrent flares as they begin ULT, and a long-acting IL-β inhibitor could potentially be of major help.

Other uricosuric medications are in development. Verinurad (RDEA3170) is a high-affinity inhibitor of the URAT1 transporter. This agent has been studied in combination with febuxostat and showed dose-dependent SUA reduction and seemed well-tolerated in an early study.[48]

SUMMARY

The challenges in approaching and managing gout are approached in four major ways. These strategies involve the entire care team for patients with gout, and active participation by the patients themselves.

The first strategy is continued education for those who care for patients with gout. Primary care physicians need to be taught, and reinforced, on the literature supporting treat-to-target for gout. Rheumatologists have a major role in this educational process. Primary care physicians need to understand that patients with gout tend to underreport their flares, and that patients with gout need ongoing support and encouragement to stay with their medication and lifestyle regimen. Rheumatologists themselves need to keep in mind that, despite optimally prescribed medications for their gout, many of their patients may be failing to adhere to their regimens.

Second, patients with gout need to be educated and motivated to help themselves and to be forthcoming with their medical providers about their gout-related difficulties and medication adherence. Patients should learn their urate goal, and learn to regularly ask their caregiver if they have reached it. They need to report their flares and to appreciate that a gout flare-free existence is a strong probability for them if they can stay with their regimen.

Third, physicians in a variety of practice settings, from solo to group practice, and from academic to nursing home to hospital practices, need to apply the people and other resources available to them to help their patients with gout. Rheumatologists in various types of practice settings can mobilize these resources to address the critical need for self-management education and adherence monitoring in patients with gout. Among the other members of the health care team who can be mobilized when available include nurse practitioners, physician assistants, registered nurses, licensed practical nurses, medical assistants, pharmacists, and social workers. Strategies for educating and monitoring patients with gout include one-on-one and group education sessions, email versus texting reminders and interactive Web sites. Online and written materials can help, but one-on-one education, especially at the beginning of ULT, is likely to offer significant additional benefit.

Finally, although the medication armamentarium for gout is presently strong, future developments can improve and refine the strategies. Pipeline medications may help to serve urate-lowering and flare prophylaxis goals with a single agent, IL-1β blockade may expand the ability to treat and prevent gout flares, and present and future uricosurics and uricase agents may improve the ability to address refractory cases. Patient adherence is likely a greater present barrier to successful gout management than the limitation of available medications, but an expanded array of treatment options will clearly be helpful.

With improved diagnosis and management, including patient education and monitoring, data suggest that great inroads can be made toward total control of gout in most patients. The major impact that gout has on quality of life supports significant efforts to optimize the available resources to the benefit of patients.

ACKNOWLEDGMENTS

The support of the Hospital for Special Surgery Academy of Rheumatology Educators is much appreciated.

REFERENCES

1. Zhu Y, Pandya BJ, Choi HK. Prevalence of gout and hyperuricemia in the US general population: the National Health and Nutrition Examination Survey 2007–2008. Arthritis Rheum 2011;63(10):3136–41.
2. Rai SK, Burns LC, De Vera MA, et al. The economic burden of gout: a systematic review. Semin Arthritis Rheum 2015;45:75–80.
3. Chandratre P, Mallen CD, Roddy E, et al. "You want to get on with the rest of your life": a qualitative study of health-related quality of life in gout. Clin Rheumatol 2016;35:1197–205.
4. DiBonaventura MD, Andrews LM, Yadao AM, et al. The effect of gout on health-related quality of life, work productivity, resource use and clinical outcomes among patients with hypertension. Expert Rev Pharmacoecon Outcomes Res 2012;12:821–9.
5. Fisher MC, Rai SK, Lu N, et al. The unclosing premature mortality gap in gout: a general population-based study. Ann Rheum Dis 2017;76:1289–94.
6. Lim SY, Lu N, Oza A, et al. Trends in gout and rheumatoid arthritis hospitalizations in the United States, 1993-2011. JAMA 2016;315:2345–7.
7. Elfishawi MM, Zleik N, Kvrgic Z, et al. The rising incidence of gout and the increasing burden of comorbidities: a population-based study over 20 years. J Rheumatol 2018;45(4):574–9.

8. Juraschek SP, Kovell LC, Miller ER, et al. Gout, urate-lowering therapy, and uric acid levels among adults in the United States. Arthritis Care Res (Hoboken) 2015;67:588–92.

9. De Vera MA, Marcotte G, Rai S, et al. Medication adherence in gout: a systematic review. Arthritis Care Res (Hoboken) 2014;66:1551–9.

10. Scheepers LEJM, Onna MV, Stehouwer CDA, et al. Medication adherence among patients with gout: a systematic review and meta-analysis. Semin Arthritis Rheum 2018;47(5):689–702.

11. Harrold LR, Mazor KM, Peterson D, et al. Patients' knowledge and beliefs concerning gout and its treatment: a population based study. BMC Musculoskelet Disord 2012;13:180.

12. Rashid N, Coburn BW, Wu Y, et al. Modifiable factors associated with allopurinol adherence and outcomes among patients with gout in an integrated healthcare system. J Rheumatol 2015;42:504–12.

13. Khanna D, Fitzgerald JD, Khanna PP, et al. 2012 American College of Rheumatology guidelines for management of gout. Part 1: systematic nonpharmacologic and pharmacologic therapeutic approaches to hyperuricemia. Arthritis Care Res (Hoboken) 2012;64:1431–46.

14. Richette P, Doherty M, Pascual E, et al. 2016 updated EULAR evidence-based recommendations for the management of gout. Ann Rheum Dis 2017;76:29–42.

15. Neogi T, Jansen TL, Dalbeth N, et al. 2015 Gout classification criteria: an American College of Rheumatology/European League Against Rheumatism collaborative initiative. Ann Rheum Dis 2015;74:1789–98.

16. Hui M, Carr A, Cameron S, et al. The British Society for Rheumatology guideline for the management of gout. Rheumatology (Oxford) 2017;56(7):1246.

17. Fields TR, Rifaat A, Yee AMF, et al. Pilot study of a multidisciplinary gout patient education and monitoring program. Semin Arthritis Rheum 2016;46:601–8.

18. Duyck SD, Petrie KJ, Dalbeth N. "You don't have to be a drinker to get gout, but it helps": a content analysis of the depiction of gout in popular newspapers. Arthritis Care Res (Hoboken) 2016;68:1721–5.

19. Khanna D, Khanna PP, Fitzgerald JD, et al. 2012 American College of Rheumatology guidelines for management of gout. Part 2: therapy and antiinflammatory prophylaxis of acute gouty arthritis. Arthritis Care Res (Hoboken) 2012;64:1447–61.

20. Dalbeth N, Bardin T, Doherty M, et al. Discordant American College of Physicians and international rheumatology guidelines for gout management: consensus statement of the Gout, Hyperuricemia and Crystal-Associated Disease Network (G-CAN). Nat Rev Rheumatol 2017;13(9):561–8.

21. Shiozawa A, Szabo SM, Bolzani A, et al. Serum uric acid and the risk of incident and recurrent gout: a systematic review. J Rheumatol 2017;44:388–96.

22. Shoji A, Yamanaka H, Kamatani N. A retrospective study of the relationship between serum urate level and recurrent attacks of gouty arthritis: evidence for reduction of recurrent gouty arthritis with antihyperuricemic therapy. Arthritis Rheum 2004;51:321–5.

23. Sundy JS, Baraf HSB, Yood RA, et al. Efficacy and tolerability of pegloticase for the treatment of chronic gout in patients refractory to conventional treatment: two randomized controlled trials. JAMA 2011;306:711–20.

24. Perez-Ruiz F, Calabozo M, Pijoan JI, et al. Effect of urate-lowering therapy on the velocity of size reduction of tophi in chronic gout. Arthritis Rheum 2002;47:356–60.

25. Baraf HSB, Becker MA, Gutierrez-Urena SR, et al. Tophus burden reduction with pegloticase: results from phase 3 randomized trials and open-label extension in patients with chronic gout refractory to conventional therapy. Arthritis Res Ther 2013;15:R137.

26. Chen H, Mosley TH, Alonso A, et al. Plasma urate and Parkinson's disease in the Atherosclerosis Risk in Communities (ARIC) study. Am J Epidemiol 2009;169: 1064–9.

27. Ghosh P, Cho M, Rawat G, et al. Treatment of acute gouty arthritis in complex hospitalized patients with anakinra. Arthritis Care Res (Hoboken) 2013;65:1381–4.

28. Ottaviani S, Moltó A, Ea H, et al. Efficacy of anakinra in gouty arthritis: a retrospective study of 40 cases. Arthritis Res Ther 2013;15:R123.

29. Jutkowitz E, Dubreuil M, Lu N, et al. The cost-effectiveness of HLA-B*5801 screening to guide initial urate-lowering therapy for gout in the United States. Semin Arthritis Rheum 2017;46:594–600.

30. White WB, Saag KG, Becker MA, et al. Cardiovascular safety of febuxostat or allopurinol in patients with gout. N Engl J Med 2018;378:1200–10.

31. Choi H, Neogi T, Stamp L, et al. Implications of the cardiovascular safety of febuxostat and allopurinol in patients with gout and cardiovascular morbidities (CARES) trial and associated FDA public safety alert. Arthritis Rheumatol 2018. https://doi.org/10.1002/art.40583.

32. Stamp LK, Chapman PT, Barclay ML, et al. A randomised controlled trial of the efficacy and safety of allopurinol dose escalation to achieve target serum urate in people with gout. Ann Rheum Dis 2017;76:1522–8.

33. Stamp LK, Barclay ML. How to prevent allopurinol hypersensitivity reactions? Rheumatology (Oxford) 2018;57:i41.

34. Bardin T, Keenan RT, Khanna PP, et al. Lesinurad in combination with allopurinol: a randomised, double-blind, placebo-controlled study in patients with gout with inadequate response to standard of care (the multinational CLEAR 2 study). Ann Rheum Dis 2017;76:811–20.

35. Dalbeth N, Jones G, Terkeltaub R, et al. Lesinurad, a selective uric acid reabsorption inhibitor, in combination with febuxostat in patients with tophaceous gout: findings of a phase III clinical trial. Arthritis Rheumatol 2017;69:1903–13.

36. Baraf HSB, Yood RA, Ottery FD, et al. Infusion-related reactions with pegloticase, a recombinant uricase for the treatment of chronic gout refractory to conventional therapy. J Clin Rheumatol 2014;20:427–32.

37. Borstad GC, Bryant LR, Abel MP, et al. Colchicine for prophylaxis of acute flares when initiating allopurinol for chronic gouty arthritis. J Rheumatol 2004;31: 2429–32.

38. Wright S, Chapman PT, Frampton C, et al. Management of gout in a hospital setting: a lost opportunity. J Rheumatol 2017;44(10):1493–8.

39. Rees F, Jenkins W, Doherty M. Patients with gout adhere to curative treatment if informed appropriately: proof-of-concept observational study. Ann Rheum Dis 2013;72:826–30.

40. Goldfien R, Pressman A, Jacobson A, et al. A pharmacist-staffed, virtual gout management clinic for achieving target serum uric acid levels: a randomized clinical trial. Perm J 2016;20:18.

41. Mikuls TR. Improving gout outcomes: the randomized evaluation of an ambulatory care pharmacist-led intervention to optimize urate lowering pathways (RAmP-Up) study. ACR Meeting Abstracts. Available at: http://acrabstracts.org/abstract/improving-gout-outcomes-the-randomized-evaluation-of-an-ambulatory-

care-pharmacist-led-intervention-to-optimize-urate-lowering-pathways-ramp-up-study/.

42. Ory MG, Ahn S, Jiang L, et al. Successes of a national study of the Chronic Disease Self-Management Program: meeting the triple aim of health care reform. Med Care 2013;51:992–8.

43. Kelley P, Whatson T. Making long-term memories in minutes: a spaced learning pattern from memory research in education. Front Hum Neurosci 2013;7:589.

44. Zhang LY, Schumacher HR, Su HH, et al. Development and evaluation of a survey of gout patients concerning their knowledge about gout. J Clin Rheumatol 2011; 17:242–8.

45. Poiley J, Steinberg AS, Choi Y, et al. A randomized, double-blind, active- and placebo-controlled efficacy and safety study of arhalofenate for reducing flare in patients with gout. Arthritis Rheumatol 2016;68:2027–34.

46. Schlesinger N, Mysler E, Lin H, et al. Canakinumab reduces the risk of acute gouty arthritis flares during initiation of allopurinol treatment: results of a double-blind, randomised study. Ann Rheum Dis 2011;70:1264–71.

47. Schlesinger N, Alten RE, Bardin T, et al. Canakinumab for acute gouty arthritis in patients with limited treatment options: results from two randomised, multicentre, active-controlled, double-blind trials and their initial extensions. Ann Rheum Dis 2012;71:1839–48.

48. Shiramoto M, Liu S, Shen Z, et al. Verinurad combined with febuxostat in Japanese adults with gout or asymptomatic hyperuricaemia: a phase 2a, open-label study. Rheumatology (Oxford) 2018;57(9):1602–10.

Moving?

Make sure your subscription moves with you!

To notify us of your new address, find your **Clinics Account Number** (located on your mailing label above your name), and contact customer service at:

Email: journalscustomerservice-usa@elsevier.com

800-654-2452 (subscribers in the U.S. & Canada)
314-447-8871 (subscribers outside of the U.S. & Canada)

Fax number: 314-447-8029

Elsevier Health Sciences Division
Subscription Customer Service
3251 Riverport Lane
Maryland Heights, MO 63043

*To ensure uninterrupted delivery of your subscription, please notify us at least 4 weeks in advance of move.

Printed and bound by CPI Group (UK) Ltd, Croydon, CR0 4YY

08/05/2025

01864742-0001